Advance Praise f

"This book contains everything that nurses need to know in order to achieve and maintain good health on the night shift. This helpful information is soundly based in science yet accessible to all readers. As a shift-work researcher and a former night nurse, I believe that all night nurses will benefit from reading this book."

–Jeanne Ruggiero, PhD, RN
Sleep and Shift Work Researcher
Assistant Professor
College of Nursing
Rutgers

"This book is a must-read for both novice and experienced nurses employed in shift-work positions. The author presents the concepts of sleep, fatigue, and health among shift workers in a relatable and thought-provoking manner. In a 24/7 world, strategies are provided to enhance health and well-being, promote work/life balance, and create healthy practice environments for nurses and the recipients of their nursing care."

–Linda D. Scott, PhD, RN, NEA-BC, FAAN
Sleep, Shiftwork and Patient
Safety Expert
Associate Dean for Academic Affairs
Associate Professor
University of Illinois at Chicago

"In *Night-Shift Nursing: Savvy Solutions for a Healthy Lifestyle*, Katherine Pakieser-Reed has provided a great resource that clearly communicates what is known about the pros and cons of the third shift. This book is an informative and insightful resource that any nurse who works or is contemplating working the night shift should read."

–Ronda Hughes, PhD, MHS, RN, FAAN
Patient Safety and Work Environment Researcher
Associate Professor
Marquette University

Night-Shift Nursing

Savvy Solutions for a Healthy Lifestyle

Katherine Pakieser-Reed, PhD, RN

Sigma Theta Tau International
Honor Society of Nursing®

The Honor Society of Nursing, Sigma Theta Tau International (STTI) is a nonprofit organization whose mission is to support the learning, knowledge, and professional development of nurses committed to making a difference in health worldwide. Founded in 1922, STTI has 130,000 members in 86 countries. Members include practicing nurses, instructors, researchers, policymakers, entrepreneurs and others. STTI's 487 chapters are located at 663 institutions of higher education throughout Australia, Botswana, Brazil, Canada, Colombia, Ghana, Hong Kong, Japan, Kenya, Malawi, Mexico, the Netherlands, Pakistan, Portugal, Singapore, South Africa, South Korea, Swaziland, Sweden, Taiwan, Tanzania, United Kingdom, United States, and Wales. More information about STTI can be found online at www.nursingsociety.org.

Sigma Theta Tau International
550 West North Street
Indianapolis, IN, USA 46202

To order additional books, buy in bulk, or order for corporate use, contact Nursing Knowledge International at 888.NKI.4YOU (888.654.4968/US and Canada) or +1.317.634.8171 (outside US and Canada).

To request a review copy for course adoption, email solutions@nursingknowledge.org or call 888. NKI.4YOU (888.654.4968/US and Canada) or +1.317.634.8171 (outside US and Canada).

To request author information, or for speaker or other media requests, contact Rachael McLaughlin of the Honor Society of Nursing, Sigma Theta Tau International at 888.634.7575 (US and Canada) or +1.317.634.8171 (outside US and Canada).

ISBN: 9781937554675
EPUB ISBN: 9781937554682
PDF ISBN: 9781937554699
MOBI ISBN: 9781937554705

Library of Congress Cataloging-in-Publication Data

Pakieser-Reed, Katherine, 1953-
  Night-shift nursing : savvy solutions for a healthy lifestyle / Katherine Pakieser-Reed.
    p. ; cm.
  Includes bibliographical references and index.
  ISBN 978-1-937554-67-5 (book : alk. paper) -- ISBN 978-1-937554-68-2 (EPUB) -- ISBN 978-1-937554-69-9 (PDF) -- ISBN 978-1-937554-70-5 (MOBI)
  I. Sigma Theta Tau International. II. Title.
  [DNLM: 1. Nursing--organization & administration. 2. Life Style. 3. Risk Factors. 4. Work Schedule Tolerance--physiology. WY 16.1]
  RT89
  362.17'3068--dc23
                        2013012102

Second Printing, 2015

Publisher: Renee Wilmeth
Acquisitions Editor: Emily Hatch
Editorial Coordinator: Paula Jeffers
Cover Designer: Rebecca Batchelor
Interior Design and Page
  Composition: Rebecca Batchelor

Principal Editor: Carla Hall
Development and Project Editor:
  Kate Shoup
Copy Editor: Clifford Shubs
Proofreader: Barbara Bennett
Indexer: Cheryl Lenser

To my husband, Bill:
Thank you for your steadfast support of my nursing career.

To all nurses who work nights:
Thank you for making a difference every night.

Acknowledgments

A book is never the efforts of one person, and this book required a team to bring it to fruition.

I extend deep gratitude to Emily Hatch, Carla Hall, and Kate Shoup for their unwavering support of this book. It truly would not have come to print without their encouragement, direction, and persistence. You moved this project forward due to your belief that this book would be an important resource for nurses who work nights.

I give a resounding thank you to the contributors of the book—to those who provided core content and to those who submitted examples of living the life as a night nurse. Your collective expertise will help many nurses (and their families and friends) understand the phenomena related to working nights. You provide excellent information, tips, and advice that will help nurses stay healthy and have full lives.

To my fellow nurses LaTonya Macklin, Peggy Hasenauer, and Kathy Hanold, thank you for your support of the idea of this book and its importance to nurses.

Three friends—Diane Rodriguez, Sharon Andrews Niemet, and Mark Zubro—have been part of my writing experiences over the years and this book was no exception. You have the ability to make me laugh when I'm in doubt and cheer me on when I move ahead. Thank you for your insight and friendship.

Finally, to my family—my husband Bill, daughter Kelly, and sons Spencer, Alex, and Patrick—you truly know what living with a night nurse is like! Thank you for your flexibility and understanding during all those years. Thank you, too, for being curious about this book—you asked questions and reminded me of stories that influenced the content of this book!

About the Author

Katherine Pakieser-Reed, PhD, RN, is the director of the Center for Nursing Professional Practice and Research at the University of Chicago Medicine. Her center is responsible for supporting nursing practice, including ensuring that nurses have access to the education and training for their roles and providing services that include the night staff.

In her 30 years as a nurse, Katherine's roles included many years of working the night shift—as a medical-surgical, intensive-care, and eventually women's care staff nurse in community hospitals and also as an educator at a long-term care facility specifically for the night shift. Katherine attributes her years of working as a night nurse as being pivotal in her development as a nurse, and believes this is where she learned the value of excellence in care, the significance of resources, and the necessity of teamwork.

Katherine holds a PhD in nursing from the University of Wisconsin-Milwaukee, an MS in nursing from North Park University, a BS in nursing from Rush University, an MA in social sciences from the University of Chicago, and a BS in journalism from Northern Illinois University.

Katherine is the author of *A Daybook for Nurse Educators*.

Contributors

Lynda Bartlett, MS, MBA, RN, is the patient care manager of the Clinical Resource Center (CRC) at the University of Chicago Medicine. The CRC is an inpatient and outpatient clinical research center that supports protocols including studies on sleep. Lynda is also an adjunct faculty member at Saint Xavier University, where she teaches the nursing care of the adult practicum. Lynda contributed to Chapter 3, "Health Issues and Prevention."

Jennifer Doering, PhD, RN, is an associate professor in the School of Nursing at the University of Wisconsin-Milwaukee. Jennifer's research studies include how sleep deprivation affects depression in urban women after childbirth and studies on fatigue and depression symptoms in lower-income urban women. She teaches maternal-infant health in the undergraduate program and research and acute and chronic conditions in childbearing families in the doctoral program. Jennifer contributed to Chapter 2, "Night Shift, Fatigue, and Sleep."

Sarah Morgan, PhD, RN, is clinical assistant professor in the School of Nursing at the University of Wisconsin-Milwaukee. Sarah is a center scientist in the College of Nursing Self-Management Science Center and with the Center for Urban Population Health Center Scientist Development Program. She teaches at the undergraduate and graduate level. Her courses include cultural diversity in health care, issues in women's health and development, and courses within the Department of Women's Studies. Sarah contributed to Chapter 2, "Night Shift, Fatigue, and Sleep."

Catherine Murks, PhD, APN, ANP-BC, is a nurse practitioner in the Center for Heart Failure Management at the University of Chicago Medicine. Her clinical specialty is advanced heart failure and cardiac transplant. Cathy's research focuses on cognitive dysfunction in heart failure and self-care ability. Cathy contributed to Chapter 3, "Health Issues and Prevention."

Mary Krystofiak Russell, MS, RD, LDN, is a senior manager for medical affairs at Baxter Healthcare. Previously, she was director of nutrition services at the University of Chicago Medicine and also for Duke University Hospital. Mary is treasurer of the Academy of Nutrition and Dietetics Board of Directors. She is the author or co-author of many papers on nutrition support. She serves on the editorial board of *Nutrition in Clinical Practice*. Mary contributed to Chapter 4, "Healthful Eating."

Jennifer Taylor, MS, BSN, BS, RN, CCRN, is special procedures nurse in the GI/IR Prep-Recovery Unit at the University of Chicago Medicine. She holds a BSN in nursing, a BS in community health, and an MS in exercise science. Jennifer has been recognized by her peers and staff nurses for her excellence in nursing. She has presented nationally on nursing care for burn patients. Jennifer contributed to Chapter 5, "Exercise Benefits."

Table of Contents

Foreword

Calling All Nurses to Invest in Their Own Health and Wellness

The health and wellness of nurses are critical not only for themselves and their families, but also to the patients for whom they care. A 2009 study found that the average body mass index of nurses was higher than that of the general American adult population. Another recent study, in 2012, found that depressive symptoms in nurses were twice that of adults in their community. Findings from research also support that nurses who work the night shift are at risk for adverse health outcomes, including high blood pressure, cardiovascular disease, diabetes, depression, and burnout. Nurses who are unhealthy and suffering from fatigue or burnout are often disengaged in their work and less capable of delivering safe, high-quality care. As a result, they, their families, and patient outcomes suffer.

Technically, cardiovascular disease is the number-one cause of mortality in the United States. However, behaviors are truly the number-one killer of Americans—behaviors such as unhealthy eating, lack of physical activity, use of alcohol and drugs, nonadherence to medications, and suicide. It would be great if all we had to do was provide nurses and patients with educational information to facilitate behavior change, but it is not that easy. Behavior change typically occurs when a crisis happens or emotions are raised—for example, a sibling dies an early death because he did not adhere to his prescribed chronic illness treatment plan. I was home alone with my mother at age 15 when she sneezed and burst a cerebral aneurysm, which resulted in her untimely death and my suffering with posttraumatic stress disorder for a few years. My mother had suffered from headaches for well over a year and finally went to our family physician the week before she died. She was diagnosed with hypertension and given a prescription for a high blood pressure medication. My dad found the prescription in her purse after she died. Who knows for sure if filling that prescription and starting on the antihypertensive medication would have lowered my mother's blood pressure and prevented her death? However, what I do know for sure is how badly I missed having her at my graduation, her being at my wedding, and her seeing my three daughters. So many people ignore illness symptoms and do not engage in preventive health care, rationalizing that they do not have time to take care of themselves and promising to start healthier practices next week, next month, or with the start of a new year.

One of the reasons many nurses do not engage in healthy lifestyle behaviors is because they tell themselves that they do not have time, given their long working hours and all their other responsibilities, including taking care of their patients and families. Nurses are great at taking care of other people but rarely take the same good care of themselves. Yet, how will our patients take us seriously when we teach them about living a healthy lifestyle if we ourselves are not role-modeling health and wellness behaviors?

Despite what many nurses think, creating more time is not the answer to being able to engage in healthy lifestyle behaviors. The solution to being healthier with a deeper level of engagement is more energy. Eating light and eating often, including three small meals a day and two to three healthy snacks; staying aligned with your life's passion and purpose; and taking regular recovery breaks (for example, spending time with family and friends, relaxing in a quiet place for a few minutes, and getting adequate sleep) are keys to sustaining high levels of energy. Aside from nurses taking the initiative to personally engage in healthy behaviors, research findings indicate that administrators and managers must create a culture and environment that make it easy and fun for nurses to engage in wellness during their shifts for healthy-lifestyle behaviors to be sustained in the workplace.

This exceptional book provides the best evidence on the risks and outcomes of night-shift work. It also provides evidence-based practices in a relatable way, along with strategies to attain a higher level of health and wellness for nurses who work the night shift. I have no doubt that you will experience many "aha" moments while reading this book and will find new knowledge that will assist you in engaging in a healthier life's journey, both at work and at home.

I will close by challenging you to make just one healthy lifestyle change today for the next 90 days, such as taking the stairs instead of the elevator, bringing healthy snacks to work instead of ones that are high in sugar and carbohydrates, incorporating short recovery breaks into your daily schedule, drinking water instead of a sugared caffeinated beverage, or taking five slow, deep breaths when stressed. Every 90 days, keep adding another healthy lifestyle behavior to your daily routine. Soon, these behaviors will become habits and easy to sustain. The health and wellness of your patients and families, and especially *your* health, depend on it.

Warm and well regards,

Bern

Bernadette Mazurek Melnyk, PhD,
RN, CPNP/PMHNP, FNAP, FAAN
Associate Vice President for Health Promotion
University Chief Wellness Officer
Dean and Professor, College of Nursing
Professor of Pediatrics and Psychiatry, College of Medicine,
The Ohio State University

Introduction

So never lose an opportunity of urging a practical beginning, however small, for it is wonderful how often in such matters the mustard seed germinates and roots itself.

–Florence Nightingale

My first position in nursing was as a night nurse in a community hospital. It was a given that new nurses started on the night shift, so I didn't think twice about accepting the position.

No one prepared me for what life as a night nurse meant. I still vividly remember the L-shaped corridor and the 22-bed layout of the unit. IVs were monitored by "drip counts"—no pumps yet for an inpatient unit. Technology was simple. Electronic thermometers were considered a luxury! What was most important, though, were the people I worked with. I was fortunate to have a wonderful manager and coworkers who guided me through the transition from graduate nursing student to professional nurse. And they helped me adapt to living as a night person in a daytime world. My peers shared sleeping tips, as well as tips on arranging my daily duties, how to handle phone calls while trying to sleep, what to eat to stay awake at night, and how to help my family adjust to my upside-down schedule.

Today, nurses continue to work with the same challenges. We continue to provide nursing care at night and will forever into the future. The varieties of night-nursing roles have expanded with changes in technology, patient conditions, and care arrangements. You can find nurses providing care at night in hospitals, nursing homes, camps, patients' homes, and even temporary settings such as clinics in buses. We handle the full range of nursing practice at night, from simple interventions to complex situations. All are nursing actions that require critical thinking, excellent assessment, often split-second decisions, and skillful application of nursing interventions.

And we provide our nursing care during the time that our bodies, by their own design, are moving against the natural circadian rhythm that would have us settle into a deep slumber. Every night, hundreds of thousands of nurses manage to overcome their natural instincts and stay awake while providing care for their patients.

So if hundreds of thousands of nurses have managed to adapt to night shift as a normal part of nursing roles and expectations, what's the concern? Nurses have shared with each other the many issues that they experience when working nights, and they have shared their tips on how to adjust to the many challenges. However, research studies about the effects of working night shifts—on a continuous, rotating, or occasional basis—finally have validated what nurses have shared anecdotally for decades. Research has raised the awareness of the risks for health care workers, including nurses and patients, and also of interventions that will help decrease those risks.

The evidence is strong enough that in 2011, The Joint Commission issued a *Sentinel Event Alert* about health care worker fatigue and patient safety, and the impact of fatigue on health care workers' ability to focus, process information, communicate effectively, and react quickly. In addition to health care providers' roles with their patients, research indicates the impact of working nights extends beyond the professional role and into one's health, safety, and overall well-being.

So, if there is information available, why create this book? The answer is simple. Night nurses asked for a single source to reference about the many issues they face—one that provides enough information to understand those issues and take positive actions. Although quite a bit of information is available about both the benefits and the challenges for nurses who work the night shift, this information is located in a variety of sources—journal and professional publications, general publications, governmental brochures and documents, organizations' communications, and personal anecdotes. However, one needs to go from source to source to create a full picture of the issues. The intention of this book is to weave together these sources of information and create an overall view of the variables that create the challenges—both as they exist individually and as they affect others—and the opportunities for improvements into one source of information. And, the book continues to keep a spotlight on what nurses like about working nights and the benefits that they perceive from being a night nurse.

This book is specifically written for all nurses who work night shifts. This includes nurses who work this shift as their standing shift, nurses who rotate to nights, nurses who pick up a shift occasionally, and even nurses who cover the shift on-call. The information is applicable regardless of the role you have—from manager to inpatient staff nurse to home health nurse. In addition, it is equally applicable to the variety of locations in which night nurses work—hospitals, emergency services, patients' homes, extended-care facilities, transportation services, and offsite telemetry units, to name a few. New nurses and experienced nurses will equally benefit from the information in this book. It is the shared experience of being a nurse and providing or supporting the provision of patient care while working against our normal circadian rhythm that makes this book's information of value to us, night nurses.

Although the book is written for nurses, our families and friends might benefit from reading it too! They will better understand the impact of working night shift. And, if they work night shift too, they will find that much of this information is applicable to any night-shift role.

This book has five goals:

* Provide a resource for nurses that brings together the research and evidence that explains the impact of working the night shift in relation to physical responses.
* Provide a resource for nurses to address the personal impact of working night shift—in particular, to our work/life balance and career development.
* Provide interventions that will decrease the safety risks related to working nights.
* Provide examples of steps that nurses can implement to improve their health and well-being.
* Provide examples of how organizations support safer and healthier environments that offset the risks for their night nurses.

The book is divided into seven chapters. Each has a unique focus, but together they create the whole perspective that nurses requested.

The chapters are written to stand on their own, but also reference where you can find more detailed information. To help you decide where you might want to start reading, a brief synopsis of each chapter follows:

* **Chapter 1: Advantages, Challenges, and Risks of Night Work.** This chapter focuses on the advantages of working nights as reported by nurses, as well as the challenges of working nights. Patient safety and health care provider risks and concerns related to night shift as identified by national and international organizations are shared. The chapter closes with a summary chart of the advantages and disadvantages of various shifts.

* **Chapter 2: Night Shift, Fatigue, and Sleep.** This chapter begins with an overview of sleep issues—deprivation, fatigue, and sleep cycle. The chapter moves on to recommendations for improving your sleep pattern and addresses the issue of night-shift napping. The latter portion of the chapter discusses the possible positive or negative impact of food, drinks, medications, and sleeping devices and apps on your quality of sleep.

* **Chapter 3: Health Issues and Prevention.** This chapter identifies the most commonly reported health risks related to working nights—cardiovascular events, diabetes, obesity, selected cancers, stress and depression, and reproductive issues—and provides brief descriptions of what may be influencing factors. Tips for improving your health and decreasing the negative influences of working nights are included in this chapter, and in the next three.

* **Chapter 4: Healthful Eating.** This chapter starts with the status of our normal night-shift eating patterns and then moves into tips and practical advice for meal options. Gastrointestinal (GI) issues are addressed in this chapter, as there is a strong relationship between the food we eat and the status of our GI system.

* **Chapter 5: Exercise Benefits.** This chapter looks at exercise from the perspective of the night-shift nurse, including benefits related to reducing health risks. Simple assessment of your current exercise pattern and response and a variety of exercise options are highlighted in this chapter, complemented by stories from night nurses.

* **Chapter 6: Work/Life Balance.** This chapter addresses the issues that many nurses talk about, but often end discussions with a sigh and little resolution. Fostering a healthy work environment through improving communication and employer support is a good starting point for establishing work/life balance. The focus then changes to what you can do in your personal life to improve your work/life balance.

* **Chapter 7: Keeping Your Career on Track.** This chapter is all about you and the steps you can take to keep your career alive and well while working the night shift. Night shift was once considered a career dead-end, but with the evolution of technology, online courses and education, and expanding roles for nurses, working nights can be converted to a significant career advantage.

In closing, my hope is that this book helps you—the night nurse—have a healthier, safer, and more satisfying experience as a provider of essential care. As you read, write your own thoughts in the book or highlight your favorite tips. Let this be a resource that makes a difference in your life. Please use this book as a starting point for having essential conversations with your peers, organization, and family and friends to help all of us find ways to improve your ability to provide safe care and to remain healthy and happy.

Enjoy the discovery! Here's to you!

Katherine

References

The Joint Commission. (2011, December 14). *Sentinel Event Alert: Health care worker fatigue and patient safety.* Retrieved from www.jointcommission.org

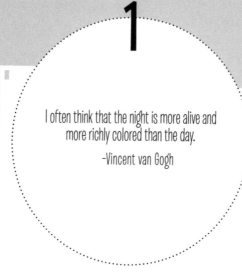

1

I often think that the night is more alive and
more richly colored than the day.

-Vincent van Gogh

Advantages, Challenges, and Risks of Night Work

IN THIS CHAPTER

Advantages of working the night shift

Challenges of working nights

Patient and staff safety

Pros and cons: A summary

The world revolves around the sun—in more ways than one! As the sun rises, so do the majority of people of the world. During the day, the world is busy. People go to work. Students go to school. Stores are open. Cars, buses, and bikes fill the road. Noise and activity are everywhere.

As the sun goes down, the world quiets down. Fewer people are working. Many return home to prepare for bed. At the same time, others get ready for night-shift work. Among these workers are nurses, who use this twilight time to prepare to go to work caring for patients.

In 2010, there were more than 2.7 million registered nurse positions in the United States. The workplace settings reflected the diversity of opportunities within nursing, including general medical and surgical hospitals (private and local), physicians' (providers') offices, home health care services, nursing-care facilities, government agencies, administrative and support services, and educational services. According to the Bureau of Labor Statistics, approximately 60%, or 1.6 million, of these positions are in settings that provide continuous nursing care (2012).

Nobody knows exactly how many nurses work nights, partially due to the variety of scheduling options that affect assignment to a night shift. Nurses can be permanently assigned to nights, have rotating night shifts, pick up extra shifts at night, or be on call for a night shift. One poll, conducted by the American Nurses Association (ANA), indicated that 35% of 1,541 respondents worked nights, and 16% worked both night shifts and day shifts (ANA, 2011, November 8). A more conservative estimate is that 25% of positions involve providing care at night—meaning there are more than 400,000 nurses working at night. And that's only in the United States!

Having a sense of the number of nurses who work nights is important. That number, 400,000, represents a population that could be a small city! The impact of this number grows when you think about the ripple effect of the care provided by each of these nurses to all of his or her patients, every night. Each benefit of working the night shift is magnified by 400,000—as is each risk.

How does one define "shift work" or "working the night shift?" Is it one shift a week? Two or more? One week out of four? How long is it necessary to work the night shift before being considered a "night-shift worker?" Conversely, how long is one considered a night-shift worker after one transfers to day shift? These types of questions make drawing any conclusions about the effects of working the night shift difficult at best (Esquirol, et al., 2011)!

Advantages of Working the Night Shift

Many people who work the night shift do so not because they prefer it, but because the job requires it (Roszkowski & Jaffe, 2012). Often, nurses who work this shift do so because they lack seniority and are required to work it (Stokowski, 2012). That said, there are several advantages to working nights, which may be why some nurses choose to do it. These include financial advantages, lifestyle advantages, improved teamwork, and more satisfying relationships with patients.

FROM THE TRENCHES

I started nursing as a midlife career change just about a year ago. I had previously been in social work and public health. When I was hired to work nights, everyone I met during my training said, "Oh, you have to get out of that as fast as possible!" Although I quietly anticipated that nights would be awful, I was also so happy to have obtained a job as an RN—especially on the unit of my choice in a hospital only seven minutes from home—that I did not want to complain.

Starting on nights was a bit rough. Adapting to four nights on and three nights off was not easy, but again, I was so happy with my coworkers, my job, and the unit that I was loathe to fuss about it. As the months passed, a day shift became available. Everyone assumed, including me, that I would jump on the opportunity to return to a normal sleep-wake cycle. I decided, however, after some hard thinking, that nights were actually working better for me and my family and that days would not be as convenient.

I work as a palliative care RN 32 hours a week. I am married, have two young children, ages four and six, and am going to grad school part time to become a family nurse practitioner. I have my hands full. Despite my initial reluctance to work nights, I found that I am able to schedule school responsibilities on my two weekdays off. I am also available, alert, and awake to pick my kids up from preschool and be the after-school caregiver. I am home for homework, dinner, and evening fun and activities.

After everyone goes to bed, I leave for work. My kids barely notice my absence. My husband does the morning routine and preschool/bus-stop drop off, and it works out pretty well. Because my children are in school, I can get some much-needed sleep from about 9:30 to 4:30 (on a good day!).

I have also found that working nights allows me to spend more time with patients, as they need my support and care. Days can be filled with chaos, and patients are busy with family or other visitors. I provide end-of-life care for many patients, and it is more satisfying to me to have time at night to help bathe, clean, care for, and support patients and their loved ones.

–Carolyn Read, MSW, MPH, RN

Financial Advantages

Often, the first advantage mentioned by nurses who work nights is the increased compensation (Andersen, 2010; Novak & Auvil-Novak, 1996; Pronitis-Ruotolo, 2001). Sometimes, the increase over the regular hourly rate is as high as 20%. The night-shift differential differs based on geographic location and how difficult it is for an organization to hire and retain nurses. Especially in today's economy, a higher income is indeed a positive incentive for those considering whether to work nights! However, it might not be considered an incentive for those who are *assigned* the night shift.

Family Life/Lifestyle Advantages

Some nurses choose to work nights because it fits with their family obligations. Often, these nurses are parents of small children or provide care for their parents (Andersen, 2010; Ruggiero & Pezzino, 2006). Depending on the family's support structure, working nights can help ensure that children are cared for by family members, reducing or eliminating the need for external child care.

In addition to being better able to meet family obligations, many nurses who work nights find that being off work during the day enables them to handle daily or weekly chores, such as shopping, in less-crowded environments. It also makes it easier to schedule personal appointments without having to take a paid day off. As an added bonus, nurses who work nights often find their commute to be more pleasant because there is less traffic and parking is less of a hassle.

Finally, some nurses simply enjoy working the night shift because they are "night owls." That is, they prefer to be awake at night and sleep during the day (Stokowski, 2012). Working the night shift is simply a personal preference for some nurses.

Working nights can make it difficult to participate in family activities and visit friends outside work. To stay connected, make it a point to schedule time with family and friends whenever possible. At the least, call them on a regular basis (Wong, 2012).

Work-Environment Advantages

When describing the advantages of working nights, nurses often talk about the camaraderie they experience with their night-shift coworkers. They report that night-shift nurses enjoy improved teamwork compared to their day-shift counterparts. This may be due to the fact that fewer resources are available during the night, causing night-shift nurses to rely on each other more (Abdalkader & Hayajneh, 2008; Anderson, 2010; Ruggiero & Pezzino, 2006). One study of night-shift nurses in Australia, where RNs and ENs (ENs are similar to LPNs in the U.S.) commonly work together, noted that "a special relationship develops between RNs and ENs during night work, because this is when both categories of staff are dependent on each other. This dependence applies to both personal relations and professional knowledge" (Nilsson, Campbell, & Andersson, 2008).

Some nurses like the night shift because the work environment at night is very different from the daytime work environment. True, the actual *workload* might not be terribly different. Indeed, there are often fewer night-shift nurses caring for the same number of patients as their daytime counterparts. But there are different routines at night. There are no organized rounds by physicians. There are few, if any, meetings. In addition, the phone rings less, leading to fewer interruptions. Also, hallways and common areas are quieter because many institutions enforce quiet zones to help patients sleep. Finally, the pace may be preferable.

Another benefit of working nights is that fewer managers are present. This leads to increased autonomy and responsibility for patient care (Powell, 2011). Also, less involvement in workplace politics is required. Because there is less competition, promotions may happen more quickly. And because fewer specialists work nights, there are more opportunities to learn and improve skills.

FROM THE TRENCHES

As a new nurse, I like working nights. The air in the hospital seems to be a little more relaxed, with all of the "bigwigs" and administrators gone for the day. It seems to be a little bit slower than day shift, as the doctors are not rounding and writing multiple orders. As a new nurse, this gives me ample opportunity to "get my feet wet," as nursing school does not fully prepare you for what it is actually like to be a nurse. Working with a good group of experienced nurses has really helped me out; they are very receptive to my constant barrage of questions, and most of all they are patient with me.

–Eric Simpson, RN

Patient Care

Night work enables nurses to practice in a meaningful way. Indeed, many nurses report that the night shift gives them the opportunity to develop more positive relationships with their patients. Specifically, working nights gives nurses "more chance to see the real person who is the patient since they aren't out at tests or visiting with family" (Andersen, 2010). There is a peace and satisfaction that comes with helping patients through the night.

Often, patients are worried or anxious during the night. Because nurses who work nights are subject to fewer disruptions, they have the opportunity to pause at the bedside, listen to patients, and relieve their worries.

Having fewer disruptions also means that nurses can establish their plan for the night and carry it through. In addition, night-shift nurses can read patients' medical records and deepen their knowledge of their patients' conditions, ensuring that the plans of care are actually what are intended.

FROM THE TRENCHES

I work nights because I simultaneously enjoy being able to spend more time getting to know my patients better, "geeking out" on all the detailed assessments and plans written by the hospitalists and consultants, and expanding my knowledge base by looking up the relevant evidence-based practice related to my patients' conditions. More often than not, it is slow enough at night that all of those are possible. And when it is busy, I am just thankful that it's not also day shift and the multiplication of new orders, admissions, discharges, and other complications that it entails. I also feel like I am a better nurse on the night shift, when I am able to give my patients the attention they deserve. Also, while I was completing my MSN, working nights afforded me the opportunity to squeeze my clinical rotations and classes in either before or after my shifts, more so than day or evening shifts (and despite the sleep deprivation that that often involved).

–Michael Bennett, MSN, RN, ANP-BC, GNP-BC

Challenges of Working Nights

Although there are definite benefits to working nights, it's not all roses. In fact, if you read any article about the advantages and challenges of working nights, you'll quickly notice that the space dedicated to the challenges outweighs that devoted to the advantages. These challenges aren't unique to any one area of nursing practice, nor are they unique to any one area of the world.

Unfortunately, this book is no different. It presents a lot of the problems faced by night-shift nurses. However, it's our view that if you are aware of the challenges, you'll be better prepared to face them, both on the personal level and at an organizational level.

Briefly, these challenges include the following:

* Fatigue
* Health issues
* Work-environment issues, including turnover of new nurses, lack of resources, and invisibility
* Patient and staff safety

Further research on the effects of working the night shift is needed, as are strategies to moderate or alleviate the negatives (Powell, 2011).

Fatigue

The most frequent complaint about working nights is how hard it is to adjust to working when the body normally prefers sleep. As a result, night-shift nurses often experience tremendous fatigue.

Nurses use many methods to cope with the disruption to their sleep cycle, some healthy and some not. These methods are discussed in detail in Chapter 2, "Night Shift, Fatigue, and Sleep."

A Sentinel Event Alert issued by the Joint Commission on December 14, 2011, articulated the impact of fatigue resulting from an inadequate amount of sleep or an insufficient quality of sleep over an extended period. The result is a number of problems, including the following:

* Lapses in attention and inability to stay focused
* Reduced motivation
* Compromised problem-solving

* Confusion
* Irritability
* Memory lapses
* Impaired communication
* Slowed or faulty information processing and judgment
* Diminished reaction time
* Indifference and loss of empathy

 Of particular concern for younger nurses (who are often relegated to the night shift due to their lack of seniority) is the fact that sleep deprivation can affect their ability to retain knowledge. As noted by Lockley et al. (2007), "Many tasks, including visual discrimination, motor learning, and insight are dependent on adequate sleep following the initial learning opportunity, and failure to sleep the night after learning a task may impair providers' ability to consolidate this learning."

Moreover, focus-group research conducted by Novak and Auvil-Novak (1996) found a high incidence (95%) of automobile-related injuries and near accidents among night-shift nurses driving to and from the workplace. (However, in its 2011 Health & Safety Survey, the American Nurses Association found that only 9% of respondents indicated that they had ever had an automobile accident that they believed was related to fatigue.)

On the topic of accident rates, a 1988 study by Coffey, Skipper, and Jung found that performance appears to be lowest between 3:30 and 5:30 a.m., as evidenced by increased accident rates in that time frame. Similarly, according to a 2001 study by Moser and Dubravec, the highest number of errors occurs at 3:00 a.m. (Abdalkader & Hayajneh, 2008).

Like the Joint Commission, the U.S. Department of Labor, Occupational Safety and Health Administration (OSHA) has weighed in on the issue of fatigue for workers—in this case, workers who work an "extended" or "unusual" shift.

Normal, Extended, and Unusual Shifts

According to OSHA, a "normal" work shift is "generally considered to be a work period of no more than eight consecutive hours during the day, five days a week, with at least an eight-hour rest between each shift." An extended or unusual shift is "any shift that incorporates more continuous hours, requires more consecutive days of work, or requires work during the evening."

OSHA notes that extended and unusual shifts can be used to maximize scarce resources and are often required during emergencies. Although OSHA does not issue standards for extended or unusual work shifts, the organization does acknowledge that these types of shifts may be more stressful for workers physically, mentally, and emotionally, adding that these shifts may disrupt the body's regular schedule. This, according to OSHA, can cause increased fatigue, stress, and lack of concentration, which in turn lead to increased risk of operator error, accidents, and injuries.

Similar to the Joint Commission, OSHA spells out symptoms of fatigue. These include the following:

* Weariness
* Sleepiness
* Irritability
* Reduced alertness
* Lack of concentration and memory
* Lack of motivation
* Increased susceptibility to illness
* Depression
* Headache

* Giddiness
* Loss of appetite
* Digestive problems

For more on fatigue and combating it, see Chapter 2.

 In its April 27, 2012, *Morbidity and Mortality Weekly Report*, the U.S. Department of Health and Human Services, Centers for Disease Control and Prevention (CDC) discussed short sleep duration among U.S. workers. According to the report, findings from a 2010 National Health Interview Survey (NHIS) indicated that 30% of employed U.S. adults, some 40.6 million workers, averaged less than six hours sleep per 24-hour period, despite recommendations from the National Sleep Foundation that adults obtain between seven and nine hours of sleep each day. Night-shift workers were even more likely to report short sleep duration than day-shift workers.

Health Issues

Apart from fatigue, there are other health issues associated with working the night shift. These include the following (Roszkowski and Jaffe, 2012; Stokowski, 2012):

* Cardiovascular events, such as heart attack and stroke
* Diabetes
* Obesity
* Certain cancers
* Stress and depression
* Reproductive issues

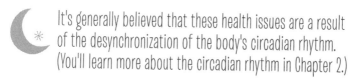 It's generally believed that these health issues are a result of the desynchronization of the body's circadian rhythm. (You'll learn more about the circadian rhythm in Chapter 2.)

For more on the health issues associated with working nights, see Chapter 3, "Health Issues and Prevention."

Work-Environment Issues

The night shift presents a few unique issues with respect to the work environment. For example, as noted by Nilsson, Campbell, and Andersson, "night duties have to be performed under difficult conditions that include working silently in dimmed lighting, and making decisions when fatigue threatens" (2008). In addition, night nurses must contend with the following:

* Turnover of new nurses
* Lack of resources
* Invisibility

Turnover of New Nurses

Many nurses begin their careers working the night shift. This can create a unique dynamic for the night shift: many newly graduated nurses with some experienced nurses. The experienced nurses typically serve both as resource and trainer for the new nurses.

Often, however, new nurses quickly move to daytime positions. This happens for many reasons: an inability to adapt to night work, general lifestyle issues with working nights, and demands of family life, to name a few. When that happens, the experienced nurses are left to train the *new* new nurse—increasing their own workload and reducing the resources available to them for their own collaboration and consultation needs.

Understandably, experienced nurses grow tired of training new nurses, only to see them leave the unit or shift soon thereafter.

Lack of Resources

For some nurses, the absence of management during the night shift helps them develop autonomy and ownership of their nursing role. For others, the lack of night managers is seen as a critical lack of resources, meaning staff nurses must handle stressful situations and make difficult decisions guided only by written policies and procedures or the advice of peers. As noted by Cochran, "It can be difficult to decide how far to pursue a concern when it is necessary to awaken administrative staff."

Nilsson, Campbell, and Andersson write, "A study about the staff's own health experiences during downsizing…revealed that nurses working alone at night felt insecure, because they did not have any colleagues to consult in situations where they had to make assessments and decisions" (2008). This can be problematic for night-shift nurses. Similarly, Powell notes that "Leadership for night staff is minimal. Nurses desire to work autonomously while concurrently expressing concern over limited skilled leadership available at night. Ineffectual leadership negatively influences worker satisfaction, morale, and patient care delivery while control over work activities has the potential to reduce frustrations and improve the nurses' outlook' (2011).

Similarly, during the night shift, there may can be a lack of physical resources, such as medications and supplies. Without management support, fixing this problem can be difficult.

Invisibility

Often, there is tension between the day- and night-shift staffs. This is generally due to a lack of understanding of each other's roles. Nilsson, Campbell, and Andersson note, "In order for nurses working at night to be fully appreciated, the communication between day and night staff in health care organizations needs to be developed" (2008). Otherwise, according to Powell, "Poor cooperation negatively impacts on patient care and worker satisfaction, manifesting in missed opportunities for patient care and interpersonal staff difficulties including serious conflict' (2011).

Some night-shift nurses believe that day-shift nurses don't understand what night nurses *do*. They believe day-shift nurses fail to see that less staff at night often means an increase in patient responsibility—not to mention the amount of work that must be done during the night shift to prepare patients for morning treatments, tests, and rounds. Some night-shift nurses liken this to feeling invisible.

Nilsson, Campbell, and Andersson (2008) note, "In the main, intrinsic value is not attached to night work which tends to make night nursing invisible. Night work is apprehended as separated from day work and night work sometimes seems to be less valuable. Night nursing is described as being controlled by plans made in the daytime and staffed with fewer nurses on the wards."

Night nurses often feel invisible not just to their counterparts on the day shift, but to the overall leadership, in part because there are few activities developed to address them on their shift. Staff meetings and other organizational gatherings frequently happen on the day shift; if night nurses wish to attend, it is often at the cost of sleep. In addition, professional seminars, which inevitably occur during the day, often require the night nurse to attend on his or her days off or even to take vacation time.

An unfortunate consequence of this invisibility is career stall, as "invisibility to daytime administrators and power-brokers increases" (Trimble, n.d.). Powell notes, "Nurses on night shift miss out on professional development. Fatigue, poor environmental conditions, and lack of designated learning time deprive night shift nurses of educational opportunities, manifesting in reduction of both knowledge and skills" (2011).

Work/Life Balance

One of the most difficult challenges faced by nurses on the night shift is maintaining work/life balance. A 2010 study by the European Commission notes:

> Shift workers are…subjected to a social desynchronization, a desynchronization from the social rhythm of a society. This means that shift workers…have to work during valuable times for social interaction and participation and thus are restricted from social participation and interaction leading to substantial social impairments.

According to the European Commission (2010), social impairments can include problems with the following:

* Effects on the shift worker's personality structure and interests
* Relations with family and friends, as well as clubs and organizations
* Engagement in public organizations such as community councils

This is especially problematic "in those domains which require a coordination of activities and where the social partners for the interaction are bound to the general social rhythm and cannot adapt to that of the shift worker" (European Commission, 2010). Indeed, the European Commission notes that night-shift workers "show a higher proportion of broken partnerships and divorces and difficulties in finding a partner/establishing a partnership," and that "children of shift workers achieve lower performance at school and have a lower chance of attending higher education…as well as showing impairments in their social lives."

Research by the European Commission is supported by that of Roszkowski and Jaffe, who note the following (2012):

A shift-work schedule interferes with activities occurring during the day, such as child care and team sports. With most shift workers sleeping during the day, they tend to miss out on important family activities and social gatherings or are often too tired to attend.

Roszkowski and Jaffe add, "The attempt to find balance between work and personal time often conflicts with the opportunity to sleep, further exacerbating the chronic sleepiness and sleep deprivation endured by the shift worker. This ultimately has a negative impact on an individual's quality of life" (2012).

Those who work the night shift must make work/life balance a priority. For more on this important topic, see Chapter 6, "Work/Life Balance."

Patient and Staff Safety

In her 2008 review of hundreds of research studies related to insufficient sleep for shift workers, researcher Ann Rogers found that individuals working nights receive less sleep than their day-shift counterparts. In addition, or perhaps as a result, people who work nights face the following risks:

* Falling asleep while working
* Cognitive problems
* Alterations in mood
* Reduced job performance
* Reduced motivation
* Increased safety risks
* Increased physiological changes

Naturally, these risks translate into serious issues with respect to the safety of both staff and patients. Indeed, the European Commission notes, "The evidence is clear: working at night bears a higher risk of an accident than during day work" (2010). Furthermore, notes the

European Commission, "there is some reliable evidence that the relative risk of an accident increases over successive shifts, and that this increase is substantially higher for successive night shifts than that for successive day shifts."

Roszkowski and Jaffe concur, noting that "the more complex the workload is in terms of task intensity, duration, and attention to detail, the greater the decline in performance and productivity as sleep-deprived workers spend more time to complete individual tasks" (2012).

Consider a pediatric intensive care unit. Patient care in a unit such as this occurs "in an unpredictable, technology-rich environment that is dependent on highly skilled providers who need constant communication—all features providing the setting for potential error" (Montgomery, 2007). As noted by Montgomery, "fatigue and excessive workload can provide potential 'holes' that may allow errors to occur." It goes without saying that such errors could be highly injurious, if not fatal, to the infants in such an environment.

As noted by Roszkowski and Jaffe, "Safety is further jeopardized during the commute home, with shift workers being at an increased risk for motor vehicle accidents, especially after the night shift" (2012). Indeed, drowsy driving is a serious problem among night-shift nurses. (You'll learn more about drowsy driving in Chapter 2.)

Pros and Cons: A Summary

Table 1.1 outlines the most frequently reported advantages of working day/evening shifts, night shifts, and rotation shifts (Ruggiero & Pezzino, 2006).

Table 1.1: Advantages and Disadvantages of Work Shifts

Themes	Days/Evenings	Nights	Rotation
Selected Advantages	Comments	Comments	Comments
Work hours and days off	Flexible schedule Days off during the week Early start and finish times	Flexibility No rotation Self-scheduling	Flexible schedule Rotation ensures fair shift schedules Variety of hours at home
Work environment and teamwork	More consistency in patient assignments More staff during daytime Continuity of patient care	Can spend more time with patients Great coworkers and teamwork Less physical workload More autonomy, less politics	Work with a variety of staff Good change of pace Varied routine in patient care Able to learn different shift routines
Sleep and circadian rhythms	Able to sleep at night Normal sleep pattern Better quality of sleep	Can sleep as long as desired Sleep better during the day No early-morning rising	Allows for more sleep Late shift allows late-morning rising

Themes	Days/Evenings	Nights	Rotation
Selected Disadvantages	Comments	Comments	Comments
Meeting family needs	Can be with kids in afternoon	Able to attend school activities	Can take off when kids are off from school
	Spouse prefers days	Can pick up children from school	Flexibility to take care of family
	More time to be with family	Able to care for elderly parent	Able to meet family responsibilities
	Easier to care for family	Always available when kids get sick in school	
Work hours and days off	Long hours, never get done in time	Working weekends and holidays	Unfair scheduling, irregular rotation
	Conflicts with children's schedules	Inflexible shift times	Frequent mandatory overtime
	Working weekends and holidays	Occasionally getting cancelled	Working weekends and holidays
	High amount of mandated overtime		No control over schedule

Themes	Days/Evenings	Nights	Rotation
Selected Disadvantages	Comments	Comments	Comments
Work environment and teamwork	Always busy, heaviest workload Always short-staffed Days do most of physical care Unit is chaotic, too many interruptions, tests No lunch break most days	Most coworkers are new graduates or new critical care RNs Difficult to contact physicians Less staff, less support staff Rare breaks, no coverage	Short-staffing No coverage for sick calls Decreased involvement in patient care planning Lack of professional involvement
Sleep and circadian rhythms	Disrupted sleep Must get up very early Sleep deprived	Awake all night Difficult to maintain normal sleep patterns, sleep deprivation Difficult to sleep during the day Messed up circadian rhythms	Sleep deprivation Change in sleep patterns Less sleep during night rotation Lots of call back when on call, little sleep

Themes	Days/Evenings	Nights	Rotation
Selected Disadvantages	*Comments*	*Comments*	*Comments*
Meeting family needs	Must leave for work before kids get up Not home in evenings with family Difficult to schedule children's needs Not home when kids get home from school	Interruption of quality family life Less time with spouse Little night or weekend time for family activities Cannot supervise kids' homework at night	Difficult to find babysitters Lack of family time Miss dinner with family See family less on workdays
Fatigue or poor health	Long hours, more fatigue Tiredness accumulates during week 12-hour day shifts are mentally and physically taxing Three days in a row are very tiring	Chronic fatigue Tired on days off Eating more and gaining weight More health problems since nights Poor diet and hydration	Shift rotation is physically stressful Constant stress, get sick more often Not productive on days off Legs hurt more

References

Abdalkader, R. H., & Hayajneh, F. A. (2008). Effect of night shift on nurses working in intensive care units at Jordan University Hospital. *European Journal of Scientific Research, 23*(1), 70–86. Retrieved from http://www.scribd.com/doc/56094884/ejsr-23-1-07

American Nurses Association (ANA). (2011, November 8). Monthly poll showed more respondents working the day shift. *American Nurses Association Nursing World.* Retrieved from http://nursingworld.org/HomepageCategory/Poll-Results/2011-PollArchive/HYS-Oct2011.html

Andersen, A. (2010, October 2). Life of a night shift hospital nurse and night nursing staff. Suite 101. Retrieved from http://suite101.com/article/life-of-a-night-shift-hospital-nurse-night-nursing-a292173

Anderson, V. V. (2010). *The experience of night shift registered nurses in an acute care setting: A phenomenological study (master's thesis).* Retrieved from http://etd.lib.montana.edu/etd/2010/anderson/AndersonV0510.pdf

Bureau of Labor Statistics, U.S. Department of Labor (2012). *Occupational outlook handbook,* 2012-13 Edition, Registered Nurses. Retrieved from http://www.bls.gov/ooh/healthcare/registered-nurses.htm

Cochran, L. (2005). A nurse manager's response. *JONA's Healthcare, Law, Ethics, and Regulation, 7*(1), 7–9.

Esquirol, Y., Perret, B., Ruidavets, J. B., Marquie, J. C., Dienne, E., Niezborala, M., & Ferrieres, J. (2011). Shift work and cardiovascular risk factors: New knowledge from the past decade. [Abstract] *Archives of Cardiovascular Disease, 104,* 636–668. Abstract retrieved from Ovid MEDLINE.

European Commission DG for Employment, Social Affairs and Equal Opportunities. (2010). *Study to support an impact assessment on further action at European level regarding Directive 2003/88/EC and the evolution of working time organisation.* Retrieved from http://ec.europa.eu/social/BlobServlet?docId=6421&langId=en

Joint Commission. (2011, December 14). *Sentinel Event Alert: Health care worker fatigue and patient safety.* Retrieved from http://www.jointcommission.org/assets/1/18/sea_48.pdf

Lockley, S. W., Barger, L. K., Ayas, N. T., Rothschild, J. M., Czeisler, C. A., & Landrigan, C. P. (2007). Effects of health care provider work hours and sleep deprivation on safety and performance. *The Joint Commission Journal on Quality and Patient Safety, 33*(11), 7–18.

Montgomery, V. L. (2007). Effect of fatigue, workload, and environment on patient safety in the Pediatric Intensive Care Unit. *Pediatric Critical Care Medicine, 8*(2), 11–16. [supplemental material].

Nilsson, K., Campbell, A., & Andersson, E. P. (2008). Night nursing – Staff's working experiences. *BMC Nursing, 7*(13). Retrieved from http://www.biomedcentral.com/1472-6955/7/13

Novak, R. D., & Auvil-Novak, S. E. (1996). Focus group evaluation of night nurse shiftwork difficulties and coping strategies [Abstract]. *Chronobiology International,13*. Abstract retrieved from http://informahealthcare.com/doi/abs/10.3109/07420529609020916

Powell, I. (2011). Can you see me? Experiences of night shift nurses in Regional Public Hospitals: A qualitative case study. Abstract retrieved from http://www.rural-heti.health.nsw.gov.au/__documents/complete-projects/final_report_dona_powell.pdf

Pronitis-Ruotolo, D. (2001). Surviving the night shift: Making Zeitgeber work for you. *American Journal of Nursing, 101*(7), 63–68.

Rogers, A. E. (2008). The effects of fatigue and sleepiness on nurse performance and patient safety. In R. G. Hughes (Ed.) *Patient safety and quality: An evidence-based handbook for nurses* (AHRQ Publication No. 08-0043). Retrieved from http://www.ncbi.nlm.nih.gov/books/NBK2645/

Roszkowski, J., & Jaffe, F. (2012). Analyzing shift work sleep disorder. *Dialogue and Diagnosis, 2*(1), 3-12. Retrieved from http://www.osteopathic.org/inside-aoa/news-and-publications/Documents/dd-3-12-roszkowski-jaffe-march-2012.pdf

Ruggiero, J. S., & Pezzino, J. M. (2006). Nurses' perceptions of the advantages and disadvantages of their shift and work schedules. *JONA, The Journal of Nursing Administration, 36*, 450–453.

Stokowski, L. A. (2012, January 24). Help me make it through the night (shift). Retrieved from http://www.medscape.com/viewarticle/757050_print

Trimble, T. (n.d.). Night shift survival hints. *Emergency Nursing World.* Retrieved from http://enw.org/NightShift.htm

U.S. Department of Health and Human Services, Centers for Disease Control and Prevention (CDC). (2012, April 27). Short sleep duration among workers – United States, 2012. *Morbidity and Mortality Weekly Report, 61*(16), 281-285. Retrieved from CDC website: http://www.cdc.gov/mmwr

U.S. Department of Labor, Occupational Safety & Health Administration (OSHA). (n.d.) Frequently asked questions: Extended unusual work shifts. Retrieved from www.OSHA.gov

Wong, M. (2012). 9 survival tips for night nurses. *healthecareers Network.* Retrieved from http://www.healthecareers.com/article/9-survival-tips-for-night-shift-nurses/169114

2

Have courage for the great sorrows of life and
patience for the small ones; and when you have
laboriously accomplished your daily task,
go to sleep in peace.

-Victor Hugo

Night Shift, Fatigue, and Sleep

IN THIS CHAPTER

Sleep science

Night owls and larks

Adjusting your sleep pattern

Workplace solutions

Night-shift napping

Food, drinks, and sedating and stimulating medications

Sleep-assisting apps and devices

Although it isn't always our preference, working nights is often the nature of the job—particularly for nurses. As a typical night shift begins between 7 p.m. and 11 p. m., night-shift workers must sleep during the day, when most people are awake.

One of the biggest challenges for nurses who work the night shift is getting enough sleep. Research indicates that "individuals working nights and rotating shifts rarely obtain optimal amounts of sleep. In fact, an early objective study showed that night-shift workers obtain 1 to 4 hours less sleep than normal when they were working nights" (Rogers, 2008). In addition to being shorter in duration, daytime sleep is often lighter than nighttime sleep "because of outside environmental noise that makes it difficult to initiate and maintain sleep" (Roszkowski & Jaffe, 2012).

The sleep deprivation and fatigue experienced by nurses on the night shift have real ramifications. As noted by Rogers, "Sleep loss is cumulative and by the end of the workweek, the sleep debt (sleep loss) may be significant enough to impair decision-making, initiative, integration of information, planning and plan execution, and vigilance" (2008). Compounding the problem is the fact that "most people are not accurate judges of how impaired they are by fatigue or sleep loss" (Rogers, 2008). Indeed, research indicates that "although performance continues to decline during several weeks of chronic partial sleep deprivation, subjective ratings level off, making self-assessment of fatigue and performance unreliable, much in the same way that occurs following alcohol consumption" (Lockley et al., 2007).

You might assume that adjusting your sleep cycle to sleep during the day and work during the night would be a simple matter. If only it were that easy! The fact is adjusting your sleep cycle is hard. As noted by Wong, "Our 24-hour sleep wake cycle is naturally programmed and wired for our bodies to wake up during the day and fall asleep at night" (2012). Indeed, sleeping while it's light out and working when most of the world is sleeping is challenging for just about everyone. Fortunately, this chapter provides a wealth of information and advice on this topic from the literature, colleagues, and experts in the field. Read on to see how *not* to lose sleep over working the night shift!

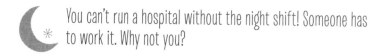

You can't run a hospital without the night shift! Someone has to work it. Why not you?

Sleep Science

Despite decades of research, scientists have yet to discover why we sleep. Some believe that organisms sleep to conserve energy. Others posit that sleep is what enables organisms to rejuvenate what is lost in the body during waking hours. What's clear, however, is that sleep is vital.

Generally, a circadian rhythm dictates people's sleep cycles. Circadian rhythms are physical, mental, and behavioral changes that occur over a 24-hour cycle, responding to light and darkness in an organism's environment (National Institutes of Health, 2008). The circadian cycle, named after the Latin term *circa dia* for "around the day," regulates the physiological and behavioral rhythms that control the waking/sleep cycle, body temperature, blood pressure, reaction time, levels of alertness, patterns of hormone secretion, and digestive functions. According to Shochat, "Under normal conditions, circadian rhythms are entrained to the environmental light-dark cycle and are synchronized with it. Thus, time-of-day effects demonstrate increased sleep propensity and reduced alertness and performance capacity in the early morning hours, corresponding to the minimum in core body temperature, the peak of melatonin secretion and the timing of the habitual sleep phase" (2012). As Smith and Eastman put it, "Millions of years of evolution have made us diurnal animals, programmed to be sleepy at night" (2012).

Sleep cycle is also affected by the homeostatic drive for sleep. This drive, which leads to an increased propensity for sleepiness, increases the longer one is awake. In addition, internal (endogenous) factors and external (exogenous) factors influence our bodies' rhythms (Marino, 2005). Endogenous factors are what we think of as the "biological clock." In contrast, exogenous factors are environmental factors, such as changing seasons, the change from day to night, and environmental stimuli or *zeitgebers* (German for "time givers" or "synchronizers"), such as noise, food, sunlight, and social and physical activity (Marino, 2005).

Finally, melatonin, which is secreted in low amounts during the day and substantially increases by evening, plays a role in the sleep cycle.

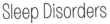

Sleep Disorders

Many night-shift workers are at risk for developing various sleep disorders—particularly circadian rhythm sleep disorders (CRSDs), described as a "persistent or recurrent pattern of sleep disturbance due primarily to alterations in the circadian timekeeping system or a misalignment between the endogenous circadian rhythm and exogenous factors that affect the timing or duration of sleep" (Sack et al., 2007).

One common CRSD for night-shift workers is shift work sleep disorder (SWSD), characterized by excessive sleepiness and insomnia, as well as increased risk for ulcers, depression, and gastrointestinal, cardiovascular, and metabolic concerns. Indeed, one study showed that 14% of night-shift workers and 8% of rotating-shift workers suffered from this disorder (Drake, Roehrs, Richardson, Walsh & Roth, 2004). Often, the symptoms associated with SWSD are completely relieved only when the patient returns to a regular, daytime work schedule. Barring that, some relief of these symptoms can be achieved through improving sleep hygiene, napping, exposure to light, use of stimulants and wakefulness-promoting agents, and use of melatonin (Salgado & Jaffe, 2012). For more on these interventions, read on.

As noted by Shochat, "Shift work imposes a continuous misalignment between endogenous circadian (24-hour) rhythms and the environmental light/dark cycle. Such desynchrony in physiological and behavioral circadian rhythms has been shown to cause sleep loss and sleepiness, and to detrimentally affect mental performance, safety and health" (2012). In other words, because night-shift nurses must fight the circadian rhythm, daytime sleep can be shorter and of lesser quality. This affects their alertness when awake and working. In addition, their total sleep over a week may be less than those who work the standard nine-to-five schedule. Finally, "The job-driven schedule of the shift worker also can affect the exposure to environmental time cues that entrain the circadian clock to the 24-hour day. Time cues, such as natural sunlight, are out of phase with the shift worker's altered sleep-wake times" (Roszkowski and Jaffe, 2012). Without conscious effort on the part of the night-shift nurse, adjusting to this schedule is hard (Åkerstedt, 1984; American College of Emergency Physicians, 2010; National Sleep Foundation 2011a; Weiss, 2004).

Night Owls and Larks

Before you tackle the issue of sleep, it's helpful to know how your biological clock runs. Often, "morning people," or "larks," adjust poorly to shift work (Roszkowski & Jaffe, 2012).

Want to know if you are a night person (night owl) or a morning person (lark)? The Center for Environmental Therapeutics provides a free, 19-question test, called the Automated Morningness-Eveningness Questionnaire (AutoMEQ), to help you determine whether you're a lark or an owl. You can find it here: http://www.cet-surveys.org/Dialogix/servlet/Dialogix?schedule=3&DIRECTIVE=START.

Research shows that regardless of whether they are larks or owls, "Some individuals are 'phase tolerant' in that after working at night they have the ability to sleep reasonably well during the day despite the fact that sleep occurs at the 'wrong' circadian phase" (Smith & Eastman, 2012). However, middle-aged and older adults are generally less phase tolerant than the young, and men are typically more phase tolerant than women.

Adjusting Your Sleep Pattern

Although some say you can't fight Mother Nature, there are ways for night-shift workers to improve sleep and circadian rhythms, as noted by Berger and Hobbs (2006) after a thorough review of the literature. Clearly, good sleep hygiene is key! Some of their suggestions, along with a few others, are as follows:

Combinations of these and other countermeasures, such as napping and the use of certain stimulants (discussed later in this chapter), are generally more effective than an individual countermeasure for improving night-shift alertness (Smith & Eastman, 2012).

*   Establish regular patterns of sleep, work, and leisure.

*   Set a permanent four-hour sleep anchor time that never varies—for example, from 9 a.m. to 1 p.m. Then add three to four hours before or after that anchor time as needed. That is, after working a shift, you might sleep from 9 a.m. to 4 p.m., but sleep from 5 a.m. to 1 p.m. on your days off.

*   Establish a regular sleep schedule when working nights and on nights off. Go to bed at a regular time—for example, 8:30 a.m. —and establish a regular wake-up time—say, 4:30 p.m. It's particularly important that you maintain consistent bedtimes and wake-up times on the shift you work most often.

*   Target your ideal wake time and shoot for it, adjusting in daily 15-minute increments. When you get there, stay there.

*   The sooner you go to bed after your night shift, the better. Your best bet is to "avoid all activities that would delay bedtime, such as housework, shopping, child care, and even walking the dog" (Smith & Eastman, 2012). Watching television may be too stimulating for some, in which case it, too, should be avoided before bed (Wong, 2012).

*   Develop a relaxation routine and sleep-preparation ritual to help you wind down. Choose a relaxation method to use in the hour prior to going to sleep—for example, reading, listening to music, or meditating (Pronitis-Ruotolo, 2001). That being said, "Avoid time-sucking activities. Choose things that you can put down when the time comes to go to sleep" (Trimble, n.d.).

*   Get enough sleep to feel rested. The National Sleep Foundation (2011b) recommends seven to nine hours, with six hours being the minimum.

* When sleeping during the day, make the room as dark as possible. Block out the light with blinds or curtains and turn off TVs, lamps, and other devices that emit light. Turn around (or turn off) all LCD clock displays. Alternatively, wear a sleep mask over your eyes to block light.

* Put away your electronics—cell phones, tablets, e-readers. Some have "do not disturb" settings that prevent incoming calls, texts, messages, etc.

 To ensure a full bladder doesn't interrupt your rest, limit fluid intake to 8 ounces before sleep.

* Eliminate potentially disturbing noises in the bedroom. Wear earplugs if necessary. Alternatively, try using a white-noise machine to drown out noise.

* Keep cool. Maintain a room temperature of 65 to 72 degrees Fahrenheit, use light bedcovers, and wear light clothing to bed. This is in keeping with the body's circadian rhythm relative to body temperature and the fact that our temperature lowers while we sleep.

 It's critical to educate your friends and family to help you get the sleep you need. Make it a point to discuss your sleep needs with family and friends. If you've opted to work the night shift to ensure one parent is always home with the children, be sure to negotiate with your spouse and children to make sure you get enough sleep. In particular, be strict about negotiating and taking advantage of overlap times (before or after shifts or weekends) when both parents are home for sleep. Also, choose social activities wisely. That is, avoid activities scheduled during your typical sleep time.

* If you awaken during your rest, get up to use the bathroom. If you're hungry, eat a light protein snack in a dim or dark envi-

ronment before returning to bed.

* Put a note on the bedroom door, "do not disturb" or "day sleeper," as a reminder to family.

 Avoid bringing stress or work worries into the bedroom.

* If sleep does not occur within 15 minutes of going to bed, get up and try again later. Repeat as needed.

 Use your bed for sleep and sexual activity only. Cognitive associations and sleep are important. See the upcoming sidebar, "Cognitive Behavioral Therapy and Insomnia (CBT-I)," for more information.

* When you wake up, expose yourself to lots of light as soon as possible—outdoor light if you awaken in the daytime or a light box if it's dark. (To find out more about light boxes, search for resources for people with seasonal affective disorder.)

* Skip the snooze button. Get up the first time the alarm goes off!

* At least three days a week, start the day with 30 minutes or more of exercise to boost your energy for the day. Stop exercising three hours before bedtime. For more on exercise, see Chapter 5, "Exercise Benefits."

* During your shift, take steps to stay focused and awake. For example, do a few quick sprints down an empty hall or perform some other types of exercises, chat with coworkers, read, or do a crossword puzzle. "Sitting idle will decrease your blood flow and cause you to become sluggish" (Wong, 2012).

* If your organization permits it, take a nap during your shift if needed. (For more on napping during the night shift, see the section "Night-Shift Napping" later in this chapter.)

* Wear dark sunglasses—preferably the "blue-blocker" variety—to block light when driving home in the morning after working nights. Research indicates that "daylight exposure in

the early morning hours…can inhibit the resetting of the circadian rhythm to match the daytime sleep schedules of night workers" (Roszkowski & Jaffe, 2012).

Assessing Your Sleepiness

Jennifer Doering PhD, RN, a nurse researcher whose work focuses on fatigue, depression, and sleep deprivation in postpartum women, recommends that all nurses screen themselves using the Epworth Sleepiness Scale (http://www.stanford.edu/~dement/epworth.html).

The Epworth Sleepiness Scale is a brief questionnaire to assess your level of sleepiness on a scale of 1 to 3 during normal activities such as sitting and reading, watching a movie, or sitting in a car at a light. Totaling the score allows you to determine whether your level of drowsiness is normal, average, or serious, requiring a consultation with a sleep expert. Bringing the results of the questionnaire to your health care provider can help to diagnose sleep problems and, ultimately, improve your health and work performance.

FROM THE TRENCHES

I am not a night nurse per se, but I do rotating shifts, as do all the nurses on my unit. I am 49, and just began my nursing career two years ago. I have found that when I have an upcoming night shift, I have to prioritize my sleep. Everyone in the family knows this! I go to bed between 12 and 1 p.m. the afternoon before, and I take a sleep aid to help me drift off and stay asleep during the day. I aim for at least three to four hours of sleep prior to a night shift. After my shift is over, I make a beeline for home and my bed. I don't run errands, clean house, or do anything distracting that is likely to keep me awake. I take a sleep aid at this time as well, read a relaxing book, and then wear both earplugs and an eye mask to keep out light. If I do not have another night shift that evening, I will set my alarm for noon so that I can get back to daytime living.

If I do have another night shift, I try to get at least six to seven hours of daytime sleep before going back in to work. I stop drinking anything caffeinated at least four to five hours before I plan to go to bed (day or night!); I find that the older I get, the more sensitive I am to caffeine.

On my off days, I go to my gym and do a vigorous workout of light weights and aerobic exercise for about 45 minutes. Then 10 minutes in the steam room or whirlpool. My gym also offers free "gentle yoga" classes twice a week, which I try to get to as often as I can. I also walk the dog a couple of times a week, sometimes jogging along, or at least keeping up a brisk pace. As a wife and mother, I find that by prioritizing my sleep and health, I am better with my family than if I am an exhausted, grumpy mom.

I also try to think relaxing thoughts, focusing on all that I am grateful for in life. I am so grateful for my home and family, who make it all worthwhile. I'm also grateful for my wonderful career, even though it requires me to work night shift! With careful planning and a fair amount of discipline, I have made it work for me.

–Anne-Marie Lillyman, BS, R

Workplace Solutions

In addition to individual sleep solutions, changes can be made in the workplace to benefit the health and safety of night-shift nurses and their patients. While it's true that we need 24-hour staffing, there are better and healthier ways to accomplish it. For example, having permanent night-shift assignments is healthier than rotating shift assignments. If that's not possible, scheduling shift rotations in a clockwise fashion, from day to evening to night shift, is more in line with circadian physiology.

Regular rotating shift workers should modify their lifestyles to allow for participation in social activities—for example, joining a health club that is open all day instead of joining a class that meets at a specific time (Berger & Hobbs, 2006).

 Administrators should educate their staff about the basic principles of circadian rhythms and the benefits of applying them to staff schedules.

Here are a few more suggestions for organizations seeking solutions (Berger & Hobbs, 2006; Efinger, Nelson, & Walsh Starr, 1995; Nursing Organizations Alliance, 2007; Ruggiero & Pezzino, 2006):

* Decrease the number of shift changes for employees, allowing better adaptability. One can adapt better with a consistent shift rather than having to alternate between nights and days.

* If possible, identify those staff members who are best able to tolerate night-shift work and schedule accordingly. Providing more opportunities to schedule shift workers based on whether they are larks or owls can help.

* Because "morningness" tends to increase with age, it might work to hire young nurses for the night and rotating shifts. It's more practical. For the most part, the night shift seems to be a young nurse's game. This isn't to say that all owls are younger and larks are older, but it seems to hold for the majority. In a 2005 review of the literature on sleep and fatigue, Muecke confirmed that the negative effects of night shift increase after the age of 40.

* Increase shift-worker job satisfaction and reduce feelings of isolation by ensuring that staff meetings, education, and development are held during all shifts. As noted by Smith and Eastman (2012), "Overtime and morning meetings should not be tolerated by shift workers, and managerial and administration staff should not ask shift workers to remain on site after the night shift ends."

* Offer shifts from 3 p.m. to 3 a.m. to prevent the bright-light exposure that occurs when night-shift workers leave for home at the end of the shift.

 Consider installing large light boxes at nursing stations and encourage night nurses to spend as much time near them during the first six hours of their shift as their workload allows. This can help keep nurses energized (Smith & Eastman, 2012). For a list of light-box manufacturers, visit http://www.sltbr.org.

* Schedule night-shift nurses for a maximum of three consecutive shifts per week, with at least two days off in a row when working an alternate shift.

* Cultivate a culture that encourages nurses to avoid working when fatigued.

* Give night-shift nurses adequate time for sleep breaks and provide a comfortable place for them (perhaps with soft music and a massage chair). Sleep breaks, or naps, are discussed in the next section.

* Give night-shift nurses access to free or affordable exercise facilities (for example, in the cardiac rehabilitation department, which is most likely empty during the night shift). This may help decrease fatigue and increase well-being.

* Reduce the number of shift-work rotations and attempt to hire more permanent night-shift workers. If the organization is unable to hire more permanent night-shift workers, use forward rotation—morning to evening to night, in that order, to go with the circadian rhythm rather against it—in two-week intervals. Research indicates that "rapid rotations and counterclockwise rotations are less-tolerated work shifts due to their adverse impacts on the quality, duration, and total amount of sleep" (Roszkowski & Jaffe, 2012).

A Word on Rotating Shifts

Research indicates that "workers on rotating shift schedules sleep the least of all alternate shift workers" (Roszkowski & Jaffe, 2012). As mentioned, if rotating shifts are your organization's scheduling preference, a forward rotation should be used, from morning to evening to night, in two-week intervals. A quicker interval will undoubtedly lead to increased fatigue among staff. "There is no way to reduce circadian misalignment for a rapid rotation that includes both night shifts and day shifts, because the circadian clock cannot phase-shift fast enough." Indeed, this type of shift system "should be abolished because of the performance, safety, and health problems it creates" (Smith & Eastman, 2012).

Several relevant organizations have also chimed in on the issue of fatigue. For example, in the same Sentinel Alert that addressed fatigue (refer to Chapter 1, "Advantages, Challenges, and Risks of Night Work"), the Joint Commission suggested actions in the workplace to help reduce the risks (2011). These include the following:

*   Assess the organization for fatigue-related risks such as off-shift hours and consecutive shift work, as well as assessing staffing levels.

*   Examine processes and procedures for patient handoffs to ensure patients are adequately protected. Handoffs are a time of high risk, especially for fatigued staff.

*   Invite staff input into designing work schedules.

*   Create and implement a fatigue-management plan. This should include scientific strategies for fighting fatigue, such as engaging in conversation, physical activity, strategic caffeine consumption, and short naps.

*   Educate staff about good sleep habits (sometimes called *sleep hygiene*) and the effects of fatigue on patient safety.

Work with your continuing education department to help with delivering this information to your staff. It could be in the form of print materials, an online learning module, or an in-person class.

* Have staff express concerns about fatigue and take action to address those concerns.

* Encourage teamwork. For example, use a system of independent second checks for critical tasks or complex patients. Although this doesn't help with fatigue per se, it does help to minimize some of the risks associated with it.

* Consider fatigue a potential contributing factor when reviewing all adverse events.

* Organizations that allow sleep breaks should assess the environment provided for those breaks to ensure it fully promotes sleep.

The U.S. Department of Labor, Occupational Safety & Health Administration (OSHA) is another organization that has taken steps to address these hazards. Specifically, OSHA (n.d.) recommends the following to mitigate fatigue when employees need to work longer than eight-hour shifts:

* When possible, managers should limit the use of extended shifts. Working shifts that are longer than eight hours often results in reduced productivity and alertness. Rather than having employees work shifts that are longer than eight hours, managers should distribute employees' hours by increasing the number of days employees work.

* Managers should plan for frequent and regular breaks throughout the work shift. If shifts run longer than the normal work period, managers should provide additional break periods and meals. Along those lines, managers should keep adequate personnel available to ensure workers can take breaks, eat meals, relax, and sleep.

Research shows that "short breaks not only improve performance and reduce subjective fatigue, they are effective in controlling the accumulation of risk associated with prolonged task performance (e.g., 2 hours sustained work) and sleepiness" (Rogers, 2008).

* If possible, workers should perform tasks that require heavy physical labor or intense concentration at the beginning of the extended or unusual shift.

* Managers and supervisors should learn to recognize the signs and symptoms of health effects associated with extended and unusual work shifts. Employees displaying these signs or symptoms—particularly fatigue—should be evaluated. Managers may opt to direct these employees to leave the active area and seek rest.

* Employees should not work extended shifts for more than a few days, especially if those shifts involve heavy physical or mental exertion.

In 2006, the American Nurses Association (ANA) Board of Directors issued a position statement on the matter, entitled "Assuring Patient Safety: The Employer's Role in Promoting Healthy Nursing Work Hours for Registered Nurses in All Roles and Settings." It reads as follows:

> It is the position of the American Nurses Association that all employers of registered nurses should ensure sufficient system resources to provide the individual registered nurse in all roles and settings with:
>
> 1. a work schedule that provides for adequate rest and recuperation between scheduled work; and
> 2. sufficient compensation and appropriate staffing systems that foster a safe and healthful environment in which the registered nurse does not feel compelled to seek supplemental income through overtime, extra shifts, and other practices that contribute to work fatigue.

The ANA continues: "Institutions that persist in policies supporting a culture where overwork, understaffing, and underpay are the norm may ultimately find themselves facing extensive accountability for their short-sightedness." This accountability may include legal implications, due to the fact that nurses' mental and physical fatigue may contribute to errors in patient care.

As noted by Czeisler and Fryer (2006), "We now know that 24 hours without sleep or a week of sleeping four or five hours a night induces an impairment equivalent to a blood alcohol level of .1%. We would never say, 'This person is a great worker! He's drunk all the time!' yet we continue to celebrate people who sacrifice sleep for work." The bottom line: It's in the best interest of nurses, patients, and health care organizations as a whole to reduce nurse fatigue.

Night-Shift Napping

Napping, particularly napping on the night shift, seems a little like *Fight Club:* The first rule of napping on night shift is you don't talk about napping on night shift! But the fact is researchers have found napping during the night shift improves alertness for night-shift workers.

For example, the National Sleep Foundation (2011a; 2011b) reports on research examining the impact of napping and caffeine on sleepiness among night-shift workers. Both were found to be effective, with a combination of the two being most effective. In addition, a 2008 article by Linda Beattie reports on a qualitative study of napping experiences, preferences, perceptions, and barriers. According to the study, not everyone found napping helpful; for those who did, however, benefits included increased alertness and energy. This carried over to the drive home at the end of the shift—a very risky time for night-shift workers.

When discussing how to improve the experience and alertness of nurses who work the night shift, people frequently mention napping. The problem is, despite support from the literature and recommendations by experts, accommodations for napping on the night shift are not widespread. Nurses do it, but often feel they have to do it on the sly. Indeed, many nurses are afraid to ask whether napping during a break is okay, and some nurses share that they help each other to nap during breaks while watching out for management.

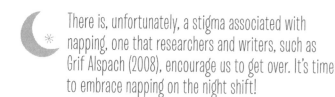

There is, unfortunately, a stigma associated with napping, one that researchers and writers, such as Grif Alspach (2008), encourage us to get over. It's time to embrace napping on the night shift!

Discussions about night-shift napping must be brought to the forefront. Organizations must establish policies that support napping, arrange breaks for napping, and offer facilities for napping.

FROM THE TRENCHES

We have a nursing retention committee at our hospital, and they continually look for ways to retain the nurses we have. One of the nurses mentioned the idea of being able to nap during the 12-hour shift. They went to the literature and found evidence that napping can be beneficial, especially for individuals working the night shift. Our policy and procedure was updated, and more comfortable furniture was purchased for the lounges on each unit. Key points from the policy include:

* *Night-shift staff are permitted to take their scheduled 30-minute power nap only in the designated nursing lounge during their shift.*

* *Each employee is responsible to begin and end their break times, returning to work alert in a timely fashion.*

* *If possible, the night-shift staff member should nap around the same routinely scheduled time frame each shift worked. Ideally, this nap time would be scheduled at the time the employee is often the most tired during their standard shift.*

* *Each employee will clean up their linens and any other refuse after themselves.*

* *Coworkers should be considerate and quiet when someone is napping.*

Nappers may bring in ear plugs or eye masks to help promote rest.

Breaks are based on patient care activity, and every nurse is expected to respond to the unit if an emergency occurs.

–Barbara Brunt, MA, MN, RN-BC, NE-BC

FROM THE TRENCHES

Earlier in my career, I worked nights in a hospital where we were given a 60-minute lunch break and required to leave the unit. They had a room on the floor with 6 to 8 recliners that staff were encouraged to use for nap time. The reason behind this forward thinking was the medication errors had decreased on nights because nurses were allowed to take a quick power nap.

–Jess Ramirez, MBA/MHA, RN, NE-BC

Naps are also beneficial when taken at home prior to a shift, 30–90 minutes before leaving for work. Berger (2006) recommends a nap just prior to going in for the night shift. That way, you'll have no more than 18 hours before going to sleep again.

Be aware that the first 15-30 minutes after waking, be it from regular sleep or from a nap, may be characterized by diminished performance, commonly called sleep inertia. "There is a transitional period between the time you wake up and the time your brain becomes fully functional. This is why you never want to make an important decision as soon as you are suddenly awakened" (Czeisler & Fryer, 2006).

Drowsy Driving

A quick nap after your shift, but before you leave for home, can be a life saver–literally. One risk associated with working nights is drowsy driving after your shift is complete. Indeed, Scott et al. (2007) found that 66% of night-shift workers reported at least one instance of drowsy driving, while 3% reported feeling drowsy when driving after every shift.

According to research, "Drowsy drivers have slower reaction times, reduced vigilance, and information processing deficits, which make it difficult to detect hazards and respond quickly and appropriately." Indeed, "Laboratory studies have shown that moderate levels of prolonged wakefulness can produce performance impairments equivalent to or greater than levels of intoxication deemed unacceptable for driving, working, and/or operating dangerous equipment" (Rogers, 2008). In the U.S. alone, "at least 100,000 automobile crashes, 40,000 injuries, and 1550 fatalities each year are attributable to falling asleep behind the wheel" (Scott et al., 2007).

Contributors to drowsy-driving incidents include the following:

* Shorter sleep durations

* Working at night

* Difficulties remaining awake during work time

If you feel drowsy on your drive home after work, the National Sleep Foundation (2011a) recommends that that you pull over somewhere safe, drink a caffeinated beverage, and rest for 20 minutes.

Food, Drinks, and Sedating and Stimulating Medications

Often, your ability to sleep and to perform while awake can be affected by your intake of food, drinks, stimulants, and sedating medications. In this section, you'll learn what works and what to avoid. (For more on food and drinks, see Chapter 4, "Healthful Eating.")

Food and Drinks

Avoid eating a heavy meal in the three or four hours before bed. Instead, eat the biggest meal of the day after waking. Protein helps with wakefulness, so is best consumed before or during the shift and not during the meal eaten before going to sleep. In addition, make it a point to eat small portions throughout your shift. This will help you to maintain a regular sugar level and will also keep you feeling energized. Complex carbohydrates such as pasta, grains, bread, and vegetables are best. Avoid foods loaded with sugar, such as candy bars, which are known to cause a "sugar high," meaning "you will feel energized and feel instant gratification, but you will crash later on. Symptoms of being 'sugar high' are fatigue, mood swings, and irritability" (Wong, 2012).

If you feel chilled, which can happen due to hormonal changes throughout the night, eat or drink something warm. (Avoid consuming caffeinated drinks, however, such as coffee or caffeinated tea, at least six hours before you go to bed. More on caffeine in a moment.) In addition, make it a point to drink plenty of water. Doing so helps to increase the oxygenation of your blood level, which aids in increasing alertness. Besides, it's hard to feel too sleepy if your bladder is full!

To aid in sleep, several medications exist. These include the following:

* **Melatonin.** Melatonin is a hormone secreted by the pineal gland and is a major controller of the circadian rhythm (Pronitis-Ruotolo, 2001). Melatonin levels naturally rise between one and three hours before an individual's typical sleep time, helping to make people sleepy. To aid in inducing sleep and improving sleep quality and duration, many night-shift workers take melatonin or melatonin receptor agonists such as ramelteon prior to daytime sleep. Indeed, "immediate-release oral melatonin, sustained-release or multiple doses of oral melatonin, and daytime transdermal melatonin administration after a night shift have been reported to modestly increase sleep quantity and quality" (Smith & Eastman, 2012). Melatonin receptor agonists have a favorable safety profile and can be used long term (Zee, 2012). Note that you should use

over-the-counter melatonin only if you are planning to sleep for at least six to eight hours.

* **GABA.** To facilitate sleep, some use gamma-aminobutyric acid (GABA), including benzodiazepines, such as flurazepam and temazepam, and short-acting nonbenzodiazepenes, such as zolpidem, zaleplon, and eszopiclone, all available by prescription only. Although they may be effective, these agents are also associated with "dependence, falls, and accidents, as well as memory, cognitive, and psychomotor impairments" (Zee, 2012). With the exception of zaleplon, which takes effect within 30 minutes and can be used to obtain as little as four hours of sleep, these medications require a seven to eight hour window for sleep. Be aware that none of these agents should be taken with alcohol (Zee, 2012).

In a recent review of literature focusing on the efficacy of herbal remedies for managing insomnia (Antoniades, Jones, Hassed & Piterman, 2012), the authors found that there is very little research on commonly used herbal remedies. Studies related to the use of valerian reflected effectiveness in improving sleep quality, but not reducing insomnia. Valerian in combination with hops appears to reduce sleep latency. Other herbal remedies, such as chamomile and St. John's wort, do not have sufficient research evidence to support effectiveness in managing insomnia. The authors recognize that many people use herbal remedies and recommend that research be conducted to assess for effectiveness of these remedies.

The U.S. Food and Drug Administration has an advisory statement on the use of kava-kava due to the risk of hepatotoxicity.

Sleep remedies should be used with great caution, as they compromise alertness, safety, and performance. It's critical that you discuss the use of any sleep remedies, be they prescription, over-the-counter, or herbal, with your primary care provider.

Cognitive Behavioral Therapy and Insomnia (CBT-I)

Another solution is cognitive behavioral therapy for insomnia, or CBT-I. The essence of CBT-I is intensive sleep assessment and training. Although it isn't a quick solution for sleeping difficulties, it is considered to be a safe and effective nonpharmacologic intervention. It includes a number of elements such as many of the sleep education and hygiene tips contained in this chapter. For more information about CBT-I, visit http://www.sleepfoundation.org/article/hot-topics/cognitive-behavioral-therapy-insomnia and http://www.mayoclinic.com/health/insomnia-treatment/SL00013.

Of course, the trick is not just getting a good night's sleep; it's also waking up—and staying up—for your shift. To aid in this, many night-shift nurses drink caffeinated coffee, tea, or soda at the beginning of their shift. Studies have shown that caffeine, one of the most widely used stimulants in the world, "improves night-shift alertness and performance" (Smith & Eastman, 2012) compared to no intervention.

Recent years have seen a proliferation of so-called "energy drinks," with a caffeine content ranging from 50-500 mg. Although it might be tempting to drink such beverages during a night shift, be aware that "the acute and long-term effects of energy drinks on health and performance are largely unknown," but that "reports of caffeine intoxication suggest that these drinks may increase problems of caffeine dependence and withdrawal as well as use of other drug substances" (Shochat, 2012).

That being said, "Ingesting too much caffeine or consuming it too late in a night shift could further exacerbate daytime sleep difficulty" (Smith & Eastman, 2012). In addition, "habitual daily caffeine consumption has been related to sleep disruption and sleepiness" (Shochat, 2012), which is particularly problematic considering that caffeine is also addicting. The bottom line? Moderation is key. "A healthy intake of caffeine ranges from two to four cups of brewed coffee a day, or 200 to 300 milligrams" (American Osteopathic Association, n.d.). In addition, "Caffeine consumption should occur only at the beginning of a shift or about an hour before an anticipated decrease in alertness (e.g., between 3 a.m. and 5 a.m.). To reduce the possibility of insomnia, caffeine consumption should stop at least 3 hours before a planned bedtime" (Rogers, 2008).

A Word on Alcohol and Tobacco

While many might think that drinking alcohol aids in sleeping, in fact, it reduces sleep latency (the time it takes to fall asleep) and efficiency and increases wake time throughout the night. As a result, "Subjective sleepiness increased, and sleep quality ratings decreased" (Shochat, 2012)—effects that were even more pronounced for women. And of course, "Beyond its effects on sleep, alcohol created hangover and reduced performance on tasks requiring sustained attention and speed on the following morning" (Shochat, 2012).

Similarly, cigarette smoking has been found to interfere with sleep. According to Shochat, "Laboratory and survey studies have reported that adult smokers experience more difficulty falling asleep and more sleep fragmentation than nonsmokers, probably due to the stimulant effects of nicotine" (2012). If you smoke cigarettes (or smoke cigars or use chew), avoid doing so before going to bed. (Of course, an even better idea in this case would be to stop using these products altogether!)

Another way to improve alertness during a shift is to take modafinil and the longer-acting armodafinil, which are FDA-approved for the promotion of wakefulness (Salgado & Jaffe, 2012). Modafinil and armodafinil, both non-amphetamine stimulants, are recommended by the American Academy of Sleep Medicine for enhancing alertness during shift work. In addition to reducing excessive sleepiness, modafinil has been associated with "small but significant improvements in performance" (Zee, 2012). Also, "fewer patients taking modafinil report accidents or near-accidents during their commute home from night shifts" (Zee, 2012). For its part, armodafinil, like modafinil, has been shown to result in "improved performance on memory and attention and reduced sleepiness during night shifts both at work and in a laboratory setting, and during the commute home" (Zee, 2012). In addition, "Armodafinil was associated with significant improvements in late-in-shift clinical conditions, wakefulness, and improvements in overall patient functioning. It can also facilitate improvements in measures of overall clinical condition, long-term memory, and attention" (Zee, 2012). Be aware that both modafinil and armodafinil are prescription medications. Your primary care provider will want to know your medical history, including any history of angina, recent myocardial infarction, and seizures (Salgado & Jaffe, 2012).

Sleep-Assisting Apps and Devices

Although putting away your electronic devices is key to getting the sleep you need during the day, there are various iPhone, iPad, and Android apps that can help improve sleep. By using some of these apps, you can evaluate your sleep and assess your drowsiness. Other apps provide relaxation exercises, help with meditation, or play white noise or soothing sounds to help with sleep.

Search the Web for reviews of apps for sleep and relaxation. Reviews may help you narrow down ones that would work for you. Searching the market specific to your device should also yield a variety of results. The following website provides information about apps for the iPhone and iPad: http://appadvice.com/appguides/show/sleeping-aid-apps. And this website lists apps for Android users: http://www.androidauthority.com/best-android-apps-sleep-insomnia-90783/. Another approach is to search in the iTunes App Store or the Android Market.

In addition to apps, various devices are available that can evaluate the quality of the sleep you're getting. Most work by tracking how often you move while you sleep. Although not quite the same as having your sleep evaluated by a sleep expert, these devices can provide information you can share with your health care provider. Searching the Web for devices for evaluating sleep quality or for sleep devices should yield a list for you to check out.

Because we love gadgets, here are some ideas to get you started if you are so inclined. One device, the Zeo Sleep Manager Pro, evaluates your sleep quality and provides coaching for improving your sleep. For more information, visit http://www.myzeo.com. They also have a sleep knowledge center and, for a fee, a sleep health risk assessment.

Another gadget that can address exercise and sleep is the FitBit. The FitBit, which is a device that you clip on to your clothing while you are awake, tracks the number of steps you take, the number of calories you burn, how active you are, and the number of flights of stairs you climb. When you are ready for bed, you place the FitBit in a holder that goes around your wrist, and it evaluates your sleep by how often you move. Check it out on the Web at http://www.fitbit.com.

References

Åkerstedt, T. (1998). Shift work and disturbed sleep/wakefulness. *Sleep Medicine Reviews, 2*(2), 117–128.

Alspach, G. (2008). Napping on the night shift: Slacker or savior? *Critical Care Nurse, 28*(6), 12-19.

American College of Emergency Physicians. (2010). Circadian rhythms and shift work—Policy resource and education paper (PREP). Retreived from http://www.acep.org/content.aspx?id=30560

American Nurses Association. (2006). Assuring patient safety: The employers' role in promoting healthy nursing work hours for Registered Nurses in all roles and settings. *NursingWorld.* Retrieved from http://www.nursingworld.org/MainMenuCategories/Policy-Advocacy/Positions-and-Resolutions/ANAPositionStatements/Position-Statements-Alphabetically/AssuringPatientSafety.pdf

American Osteopathic Association. (n.d.). Making healthy caffeine habits. *American Osteopathic Association.* Retrieved from http://www.osteopathic.org/osteopathic-health/about-your-health/health-conditions-library/general-health/Pages/caffiene.aspx

Antoniades, J., Jones, K., Hassed, C., & Piterman, L. (2012). Sleep. . .naturally: A review of the efficacy of herbal remedies for managing insomnia. *Alternative and Complementary Therapies, 18*(3), 136-140.

Beattie, L. (2008). Study finds nurses need their naps. *NurseZone.com.* Retrieved from http://www.nursezone.com/nursing-news-events/more-news/Study-Finds-Nurses-Need-Their-Naps_28834.aspx

Berger, A., & Hobbs, B. (2006). Impact of shift work on the health and safety of nurses and patients. *Clinical Journal of Oncology Nursing, 10*(4), 465-471.

Center for Environmental Therapeutics. (n.d.). The Automated Morningness-Eveningness Questionnaire. Retrieved from http://www.cet.org

Czeisler, C., & Fryer, B. (2006). Sleep deficit: The performance killer. *Harvard Business Review*. Retrieved from http://hbr.org/2006/10/sleep-deficit-the-performance-killer

Drake, C. L., Roehrs, T., Richardson, G., Walsh, J. K., & Roth, T. (2004). Shift work sleep disorder: Prevalence and consequences beyond that of symptomatic day workers. *Sleep, 27*(8), 1453–1462.

Efinger, J., Nelson, L., & Walsh Starr, J. (1995). Understanding circadian rhythms: A holistic approach to nurses and shift work. *Journal of Holistic Nursing, 13*(4), 306-322.

Lally, R. M. (2009, March). Badge of honor or recipe for disaster: The importance of adequate sleep for nurses. *ONS Connect, 24*(3), e-12.

Lockley, S. W., Barger, L. K., Ayas, N. T., Rothschild, J. M., Czeisler, C. A., & Landrigan, C. P. (2007). Effects of health care provider work hours and sleep deprivation on safety and performance. *Joint Commission Journal on Quality and Patient Safety, 33*(11), 7–18. Retrieved from http://www.ncbi.nlm.nih.gov/pubmed/18173162

Marino, P. C. (2005). Biological rhythms as a basis for mood disorders. Retrieved from http://www.personalityresearch.org/papers/marino.html

Muecke, S. (2005). Effects of rotating night shifts: Literature review. *Journal of Advanced Nursing, 50*(4), 433-439.

National Institutes of Health. (2008). Circadian rhythms fact sheet. Retrieved from http://www.nigms.hih.gov/Education/Factsheet_CircadianRhythms.htm?wvsessionid=wv6b1e07b629d45b6a3f20bd379566f4e

National Sleep Foundation. (2011a). Napping / National Sleep Foundation—Information on sleep health and safety. *The National Sleep Foundation*. Retrieved from www.sleepfoundation.org/article/sleep-topics/napping

National Sleep Foundation. (2011b). How much sleep do we really need? / National Sleep Foundation—Information on sleep health and safety. *The National Sleep Foundation*. Retrieved from www.sleepfoundation.org/article/how-sleep-works/how-much-sleep-do-we-really-need

Nursing Organizations Alliance. (2007). Principles of fatigue that impact safe nursing practice. Retrieved from http://ana.nursingworld.org/position/fatigueprin

Pronitis-Ruotolo, D. (2001). Surviving the night shift: Making Zeitgeber work for you. *American Journal of Nursing, 101*(7), 63–68.

Rogers, A. (2008). The effects of fatigue and sleepiness on nurse performance and patient safety. In R. G. Hughes (Ed.), *Patient safety and quality: An evidence-based handbook for nurses*. (AHRQ Publication No. 08-0043). Retrieved from http://www.ncbi.nlm.nih.gov/books/NBK2645/

Roszkowski, J., & Jaffe, F. (2012). Analyzing shift work sleep disorder. *Dialogue and Diagnosis, 2*(1), 3-12. Retrieved from http://www.osteopathic.org/inside-aoa/news-and-publications/Documents/dd-3-12-roszkowski-jaffe-march-2012.pdf

Ruggiero, J. S., & Pezzino, J. M. (2006). Nurses' perceptions of the advantages and disadvantages of their shift and work schedules. *Journal of Nursing Administration, 36*(10), 450-453.

Sack, R. L., Auckely, D., Carskadon, M. A., Wright, K. P., Jr., Vitello, M. V., & Zhdanova, I. V. (2007). Circadian rhythm sleep disorders: Part I, Basic principles, shift work and jet lag disorders. *Sleep, 30*(11), 1460–1483.

Salgado, G., & Jaffe, F. (2012). Treatments of patients with shift work sleep disorder. *Dialogue and Diagnosis, 2*(1), 27-32. Retrieved from http://www.osteopathic.org/in-side-aoa/news-and-publications/Documents/dd-27-32-salgado-jaffe-march-2012.pdf

Scott, L. D., Hwang, W., Rogers, A. E., Nysse, T., Dean, G. E., & Dinges, D. F. (2007). The relationship between nurse work schedules, sleep duration, and drowsy driving. *Sleep, 30*(12), 1801–1807.

Shochat, T. (2012). Impact of lifestyle and technology developments on sleep. *Nature and Science of Sleep, 2012*(4), 19–31. Retrieved from http://www.dovepress.com/impact-of-lifestyle-and-technology-developments-on-sleep-peer-reviewed-article-NSS

Smith, M. R., & Eastman, C. I. (2012). Shift work: Health, performance and safety problems, traditional countermeasures, and innovative management strategies to reduce circadian misalignment. *Nature and Science of Sleep, 2012*(4), 111–132.

The Joint Commission. (2011, December 14). *Sentinel Event Alert: Health care worker fatigue and patient safety.* Retrieved from http://www.jointcommission.org/assets/1/18/sea_48.pdf

Trimble, T. (n.d.). Night shift survival hints. *Emergency Nursing World.* Retrieved from http://enw.org/NightShift.htm

U.S. Department of Labor, Occupational Safety & Health Administration (OSHA). (n.d.). Frequently asked questions: Extended unusual work shifts. Retrieved from http://www.osha.gov/OshDoc/data_Hurricane_Facts/faq_longhours.html

Weiss, B. (2004). Balancing act: Taking on the night shift. *RN, 67*(8), 59-60.

Wong, M. (2012). 9 survival tips for night shift nurses. *healthecareers Network.* Retrieved from http://www.healthecareers.com/article/9-survival-tips-for-night-shift-nurses/169114

Zee, P. (2012). Struggling with shift work disorder. *Medscape Education.* Retrieved from http://www.medscape.org/viewarticle/769403_12

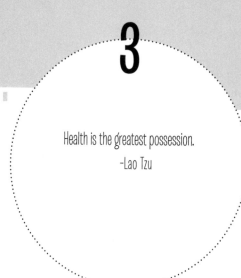

3

Health is the greatest possession.
-Lao Tzu

Health Issues and Prevention

IN THIS CHAPTER

Cardiovascular events

Diabetes

Obesity

Cancer

Stress and depression

Reproductive issues

General tips for healthy living

If the number of studies conducted to ascertain the hazards of working nights—something that's increasingly common in our 24-hour society—is any indicator, the health consequences of working night shifts are significant indeed. Results of these studies differ with respect to the consequences of working the night shift on health, but despite the contradictions, "Many of the negative health outcomes associated with working nights are considered biologically plausible" (Stokowski, 2012). Specifically, night-shift nurses and other late-night workers may be faced with increased risk for the following:

* Cardiovascular events, such as heart attack and stroke
* Diabetes
* Obesity
* Certain cancers
* Stress and depression
* Reproductive issues

Why, exactly, might working nights take a toll on one's health? No one can say for sure. However, research suggests that "sleep deprivation and circadian dysynchrony are involved in changes in neuroendocrine function, reduced capacity of the immune system, metabolic disturbances and tumor growth" (Shochat, 2012). In addition, "Exposure to light at night, leading to melatonin suppression, has also been implicated as an underlying mechanism" (Shochat, 2012).

Although working the night shift can take a toll on a healthy person's overall well-being, it is also important to recognize that if you have a medical condition already, such as diabetes or hypertension, working the night shift may compromise your ability to care for your condition. If you take medications, for example, working nights may make it difficult to manage doses of your medications. Certain medications, such as diuretics, may be problematic when working a busy unit. Medications that are timed around meals may also pose a problem, as the requirements of the unit may not allow you to eat on a predetermined schedule. If these or other issues become problematic, discuss alternatives with your primary care provider and adapt accordingly.

Working the night shift may also make it more difficult to participate in self-management activities such as visiting your primary care provider, following a special diet, or exercising. If any of these things become problematic, discuss it with your care provider and work together to develop reasonable solutions. You can also reach out to your occupational medicine department for a solution.

Cardiovascular Events

Research has revealed that night-shift workers have a higher risk for cardiovascular events, such as heart attack, stroke, or other coronary events, than their day-shift counterparts (Bogglid & Knutsson, 1999; Kawachi et al., 1995; Vyas et al., 2012). Indeed, "Shift workers were estimated to have a 40% increased risk for cardiovascular disease" (Bercz & Jaffe, 2012). Another study demonstrated that night-shift workers were 23% more likely to have a heart attack and 5% more likely to suffer a stroke (Mann, 2012).

Exactly why this is so is not well known. Here are a few possibilities:

* **Obesity.** Obesity is a strong risk factor for development of cardiovascular disease. Many studies have demonstrated that night-shift workers have a higher prevalence of obesity than day-shift workers (Esquirol et al., 2011).

* **Increased triglyceride levels.** Many studies have demonstrated an increase in triglyceride levels in night-shift workers, thereby increasing the risk for cardiovascular events (Esquirol et al., 2011).

* **Increased homocysteine.** Current literature suggests that levels of homocysteine, an amino acid found in the blood, are increased in night-shift workers compared to their daytime colleagues, putting them at greater risk for cardiovascular disease (Esquirol et al., 2011).

* **Metabolic syndrome.** It is believed that night-shift workers are more likely to suffer from metabolic syndrome than day-shift workers (Esquirol, et al., 2011), putting them at increased

risk for cardiovascular disease. Metabolic syndrome is a constellation of risk factors that includes increased waist size, hypertension, glucose and lipid derangements, and inflammatory and thrombotic states (Grundy, Brewer, Cleeman, Smith, & Lenfant, 2004).

FROM THE TRENCHES

I have noticed some adverse health effects in myself. Despite being a strict vegetarian with a pretty healthy primarily organic diet, I have noticed an upward trend in my total cholesterol from my blood donation reports. Although I haven't been formally diagnosed, I can see how one might develop a lipid disorder simply by working night shift, given what I know about cholesterol metabolism. But I suppose I must admit my reliance upon energy bars for quick nutrition and energy during busy shifts (a habit that I've since abandoned) might have contributed.

–Michael Bennett, MSN, RN, ANP-BC, GNP-BC

* **Hypertension.** Yet another risk factor for cardiovascular disease is hypertension, which is more common among night-shift workers—particularly those who have worked this shift for longer periods of time—than workers on the day shift (Esquirol, et al., 2011). Long known to be a powerful risk factor for cardiovascular disease, it is also considered highly modifiable and likely significant in terms of decreasing cardiovascular risk when well controlled.

African Americans seem to be disproportionately affected by working the night shift, with African-American women who have worked the night shift having a 46% higher risk of developing hypertension than those who never worked the night shift (Lieu, Curhan, Schernhammer, & Forman, 2011).

* **Smoking.** It is important to remember the effect of smoking on cardiovascular health. Arguably the single biggest health hazard in the United States today, smoking increases a person's risk of not only acquiring heart disease, but also cancer, hypertension, lung disease, diabetes, and periodontal disease. Still, night-shift workers are more likely to smoke than day-shift workers and are more likely to start smoking while working the night shift than day-shift workers (Esquirol, et al., 2011).

* **Stress.** Recently, attention has turned to the idea of stress and the role it plays in cardiovascular health for night-shift workers. Scientists have long recognized the effect of stress on cardiovascular disease, but only recently has a link been made to the types of stress imposed on night-shift workers. The problems associated with stress for night-shift workers are discussed in more detail later in this chapter.

Sounds pretty dismal, doesn't it? The good news is that many of the risk factors leading to cardiovascular disease are reversible by simply adopting healthy habits, such as following a heart-healthy diet (discussed in Chapter 4, "Healthful Eating") and getting regular exercise. In addition, quitting smoking can have a considerable benefit. Finally, managing stress is key to staving off cardiovascular events.

Screening for cardiovascular conditions is also important. Annual routine checkups should include a simple screening for risk of cardiovascular events. In addition, family history of cardiovascular disease is an important factor to consider when determining someone's overall risk for cardiovascular events. Know your overall risk for cardiovascular events and speak with your health care provider about screening tests that may prove beneficial for you.

Finally, it is imperative that you be aware of signs and symptoms of cardiovascular events such as stroke or heart attack and seek medical attention immediately if they occur. Heart-attack symptoms may not always be the classic chest pain or pressure followed by clutching of the chest commonly depicted on television or in movies. Particularly in women, heart-attack symptoms are less clear and often mistaken for depression, fatigue, gastroesophageal reflux, or hypochondria. If you are unduly fatigued or nauseated, or experience indigestion, shortness of breath, weakness, sweating, or shoulder or back pain, seek medical attention, as you could be having a heart attack. More often than not, symptoms of heart attack in women are less severe than those in men (McSweeney, Cody, & Crane, 2001; McSweeney, Cody, O'Sullivan, Elbersol, Moser, & Garvin, 2003). Similarly, if you experience numbness or weakness in your arms or legs (particularly if on only one side of the body), a facial droop, difficulty speaking, confusion, loss of balance, temporary blindness in part or all of your eye, or a severe headache, seek medical attention, as these could be signs of stroke. With either of these conditions, time is of the essence. A delay in treatment could mean debilitating loss of heart or brain function for life.

Diabetes

Recent research has shown that women who work rotating night shifts are more likely to develop type 2 diabetes—a disease that, over time, can damage vital organs including kidneys, nerves, and the heart—than women working a regular schedule (Pan, Schernhammer, Sun & Hu, 2011). Furthermore, the longer women work a rotating shift schedule, as with hypertension, the greater the risk of developing type 2 diabetes. Indeed, women who had engaged in shift work for 20 or more years had a 44% increased risk of developing type 2 diabetes, even after adjusting for body mass index (BMI), which is a known contributor to the development of type 2 diabetes (Pan et al., 2011).

Whether their diabetes is a product of their shift work or an existing condition, "it appears certain that regular food intake and appropriate timing of medications can be challenging for individuals with diabetes mellitus who are engaged in shift work, and this challenge may lead to impaired blood sugar control and a greater burden of diabetic complications" (Bercz & Jaffe, 2012).

As with cardiovascular disease, there is no single cause, but rather several factors contributing to this risk. Diabetes is often tied to obesity (more prevalent among night-shift workers than their daytime counterparts) and metabolic syndrome (again, believed to be more common among those who work the night shift). Smoking—a habit in which more night-shift workers partake than their daytime counterparts, as previously discussed (Gordon, 2011)—is also a factor. In addition, the association between diabetes and night-shift work may relate to the chronic misalignment of the circadian rhythm common among night-shift workers, discussed in Chapter 2, "Night Shift, Fatigue, and Sleep." According to researchers, this misalignment can trigger a decrease in leptin and an increase in glucose and insulin (Pan et al., 2011), all hallmarks of type 2 diabetes. Finally, sleep deprivation may also be a factor. Research has shown that "the relative risk of developing diabetes with persistent sleep of short durations (5 to 6 hours or fewer per night) is 1.28" (Zee, 2012).

Fortunately, as with cardiovascular disease, you can reverse many of the risk factors leading to diabetes by adopting healthy habits, such as following a heart-healthy diet, getting regular exercise, quitting smoking, and losing weight if you are overweight.

According to the American Diabetes Association (2002), health care providers should consider screening for diabetes with a simple fasting blood glucose test every three years in individuals older than 45 years. For individuals at greater risk of diabetes, screening may begin at a younger age and/or be performed more frequently.

Risk factors for diabetes include the following:

* Persons with a family history of diabetes
* Persons over 45 years of age
* Persons who are overweight
* Persons with poor glucose metabolism
* Persons who do not participate in regular exercise
* Persons with high blood pressure or lipid abnormalities
* Persons of African American, Hispanic or Latino, Asian, Pacific Islander, or American Indian races or ethnicities

* Women who had pregnancy-induced diabetes or who delivered an infant weighing nine pounds or more at birth

Of course, if you have symptoms of diabetes, such as polyuria, polydipsia, polyphagia, weight loss, fatigue, frequent infections, trouble with your vision, or sores or wounds that don't heal, consult your health care provider immediately.

Obesity

Obesity is defined by the Centers for Disease Control and Prevention (CDC) and the World Health Organization (WHO) as a body mass index (BMI) of greater than 30. (Those with a BMI of 25–29.9 are considered overweight.) With obesity come a host of detrimental comorbidities, including hypertension, diabetes, lipid disorders, cardiovascular disease, liver and gallbladder disease, and cancer (Eberly & Feldman, 2010).

Calculating BMI

To calculate your BMI, use this formula:

$$\text{Weight (lb)} / [\text{Height (in)}]^2 \times 703$$

So, for example, a person who weighs 160 lbs and stands 68 inches tall would have a BMI of 24.325:

$$160 \text{ lb} / [68 \text{ in}]^2 \times 703 = 24.325$$

Unfortunately, it appears that night-shift workers are particularly prone to obesity. According to one study of 85 employees in a New York City hospital, late-shift workers (evening and night shifts) experienced more weight gain than did day workers since beginning their respective shifts. A different study observed "a trend of increasing BMI with increasing duration of night-shift work (spanning 1 to 15+ years)" (Eberly & Feldman, 2010). Indeed, according to Eberly and Feldman,

"Shift work appears to be an independent risk factor for obesity in addition to the more widely recognized factors of age, gender, race, diet, level of physical activity, family history of obesity, and socioeconomic status" (2010).

 Talk with your health care provider or with a registered dietitian about the best weight for you so you can reduce your chances of developing heart disease, diabetes, and even some cancers. Contrary to current belief, you do not need to be stick thin!

Why does working night shift contribute to increased weight? It seems the answer is still being unraveled. Do nurses who weigh more prefer to work the night shifts? While this hardly seems likely, many biological theories do exist to explain the relationship between working nights and weight gain. One such theory, supported by a growing body of evidence, is that sleep duration is "linked to metabolism and the regulation of appetite" (Rogers, 2008). In other words, people who get inadequate quality sleep—common among night-shift workers— are more prone to gain weight. According to Zee (2012), 924 adults in a primary care practice who were overweight or obese slept less than adults with normal BMIs. Eberly and Feldman (2010) describe another study that revealed that "increased BMI was proportional to decreased sleep in those with less than 8 hours of sleep. The lowest measured BMI was found in those who slept an average of 7.7 hours." They propose a biological basis to this weight gain, going on to explain, "Shorter sleep duration was associated with lower levels of leptin, which suppresses appetite, and increased levels of ghrelin, which increases appetite" (2010).

Further complicating matters for night-shift workers is the circadian rhythm, or rather, disruptions in the circadian rhythm. As you learned in Chapter 2, a circadian rhythm dictates people's sleep cycles and controls their body temperature, blood pressure, reaction time, levels of alertness, patterns of hormone secretion, and digestive function. Normally, digestive processes slow in the evening and overnight. If this rhythm is interrupted by shift work, when you eat may be out of sync with the normal digestive slowing in the evening and night. As a result, your body may not be able to process what you eat efficiently, leading to weight gain. This theory is supported in a 2009 study by Arble, Bass, Laposky, Vitaterna, and Turek, which explored the role of the circadian phase of food consumption in weight gain. This study found that mice who were fed contrary to their circadian rhythm (in their case during the day, as they are typically nocturnal) weighed significantly more after a six-week period than mice who were fed roughly the same amount during the "right" feeding time. According to researchers, these results could easily translate to humans, explaining the relationship between shift work and weight gain.

Although some of the differences in weight may be explained by time, the amount of food consumption should also be considered. In one study, "Night workers reported an increase in food intake, later last daily meal times, more and longer naps, and less exercise, all of which may have contributed to greater weight gain" (Eberly & Feldman, 2010). In another study, this one by Persson and Martensson, "Many of the nurses reported eating foods high in sugar in order to override the feeling of tiredness. Sweet foods and junk food were readily consumed due to ease of access compared to an alternatively healthy snack" (2006).

Finally, it is also important to consider the effect of exercise. It has been observed that people who get inadequate quality sleep (again, common among night-shift workers) lack the energy to engage in physical activity. Unfortunately, Eberly and Feldman note, "This can be a vicious cycle difficult to break if not addressed quickly. Exercise energizes the body. Clearly, individuals who do not exercise do not benefit from the energy provided, and therefore continue in their feeling of lassitude" (2010).

Eberly and Feldman offer several suggestions for night-shift workers who seek to avoid obesity (2010):

* Limit the number of shifts worked in a row to four, followed by at least 48 consecutive hours off. This helps to limit sleep deprivation, and by extension, weight gain.

* Make sleep a priority and follow good sleep hygiene. (For more information, refer to Chapter 2.)

* Eat nutritious foods (think fruits and vegetables) while working. This helps prevent fluctuations in glucose levels. (For more on healthy eating, see Chapter 4.)

* Exercise! This both energizes the body, helping to combat fatigue, and burns calories, helping to prevent weight gain. Note, however, that exercise should be avoided just before bedtime, as its energizing effects may make sleep difficult. (For more on exercising, see Chapter 5, "Exercise Benefits.")

* Take advantage of employer-based wellness programs, if available. According to Eberly and Feldman, "A number of studies have shown that employer-based wellness programs can be beneficial to employees and can be cost effective for the employer" (2010).

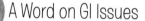

A Word on GI Issues

Perhaps due to disruption to the circadian rhythm, which causes alterations in the secretion of leptin and ghrelin (which are responsible for the regulation of satiety and appetite, respectively), or possibly because they lack easy access to nutritious meals, some 50% of permanent night-shift workers grapple with appetite disturbances or gastrointenstinal problems (Bercz & Jaffe, 2012). You'll learn more about these in Chapter 4.

Cancer

In 2007, the International Agency for Research on Cancer (IARC), part of the World Health Organization (WHO), classified shift work involving circadian rhythm disruption as a group-2A carcinogen, meaning, according to Bercz and Jaffe, that "there is limited evidence of carcinogenicity in humans but sufficient evidence of carcinogenicity in experimental animals" (2012). Of particular concern for night-shift workers are breast (women), prostate (men), and colorectal cancers.

The reasons for the IARC classification may pertain at least in part to circadian rhythm disruption—in particular, the reduced secretion of the hormone melatonin, which is known to have both direct and indirect tumor-suppressing properties (Bercz & Jaffe, 2012). In addition, according to Bercz and Jaffe, "Changes in melatonin secretion also cause the phenomenon of phase shift, in which loss of synchrony occurs between rhythmic bodily functions and the sleep/wake cycle. This loss, in turn, is thought to alter the control of cell and tissue proliferation" (2012). Other factors include disturbances of reproductive hormones and the stress-related secretion of cortisol and the resultant depression of immune function (Bercz & Jaffe, 2012). Bercz and Jaffe also note that "reduced vitamin D production and lifestyle changes associated with shift work (but not necessarily with circadian rhythm disruption) may also play roles" (2012).

Breast Cancer

Breast cancer, the most common type of cancer in women, is unlike most other forms of common cancers in that its major cause is unknown. That is, as noted by researcher Richard G. Stevens, "There is scientific consensus that the bulk of lung cancer cases is explained by smoking, of liver cancer by hepatitis viruses and aflatoxin, of cervical cancer by human papilloma virus, of stomach cancer by *Helicobacter pylori* and much of colon cancer by family history, physical activity and diet. For breast cancer there is no consensus on the major causes, and it thus remains a mystery" (2009).

One theory, as noted by Stevens, is that "a portion of the breast cancer burden might be explained by the introduction and increasing use of electricity to light the night" (2009). The so-called "light-at-night," or "LAN," theory posits that exposure to electric light at night "would lower melatonin production by the pineal gland, and that this suppression of melatonin might then lead to increased breast cancer risk by leading to increased oestrogen production" (Stevens, 2009). Stevens also notes that "LAN may also disrupt cortisol rhythms, and that may affect breast cancer risk and/or prognosis" (2009). Finally, according to Stevens, lack of exposure to sunshine (and the resulting inadequate production of vitamin D) could be a factor. Naturally, if the LAN theory is correct, night-shift workers would be at higher risk for the disease.

Various studies have indeed shown that night-shift workers are at higher risk for breast cancer. One study of 18,551 female military employees, conducted in Denmark, "found that any night work increased the adjusted odds of breast cancer by 40% vs. never working nights. The study also determined that the risk appeared to increase with longer duration of intense night shifts" (Zee, 2012). Whether the cause is due to night-shift workers' frequent exposure to electric light at night, circadian rhythm disruption, sleep deprivation, lack of exposure to sunlight, a combination of these, or something else entirely remains unclear. As such, it's difficult to know what preventive measures to take beyond the basics, such as eating healthfully and exercising. (On the topic of exercising, research has shown that those who engaged in vigorous physical activity—jogging, running, bicycling, swimming, tennis and/or squash, calisthenics, aerobics, or using a rowing machine—were 20% less likely to contract breast cancer [Bumgardner, 2008].) And of course, regular self exams and mammograms are critical for night-shift workers due to their increased risk.

Colorectal Cancer

Data from the Nurses' Health Study has revealed that women who work three or more night shifts per month for 15 years or more face a 35% increased risk of colorectal cancer (Bercz & Jaffe, 2012). It's not yet known whether men who work the night shift face an increased risk for this disease, but as noted by Bercz and Jaffe, "it is plausible to assume that male shift workers could be at an even higher risk given the already increased colon cancer risk among men" (2012).

As with the other cancers discussed in this section, colorectal cancer among night-shift workers is likely caused by circadian rhythm disruption—in particular, the reduced secretion of melatonin (Schernhammer et al., 2003). In the case of intestinal cancers, the reduction of melatonin affects the growth of cell lines derived from hormone-independent carcinomas. In addition, "the finding that colorectal cancer patients had lower plasma levels of melatonin than healthy control subjects suggests a possible link between low melatonin levels and the enhanced development of colorectal cancer in humans" (Schernhammer et al., 2003).

According to the American Cancer Society (ACS; 2013), you can reduce your risk for colon cancer by eating more vegetables, fruits, and whole grains, and by reducing your intake of red meat and processed meat. Alcohol intake should be limited to at most two drinks per day for men and one drink per day for women. Of course, exercising, maintaining a healthy weight, and refraining from smoking all reduce your risk for colon cancer.

The signs and symptoms of colorectal cancer according to the ACS (2013) include the following:

* A change in bowel habits, such as diarrhea, constipation or narrowing of the stool, that lasts for more than a few days
* A feeling that you need to have a bowel movement, but are not relieved by doing so
* Rectal bleeding, dark stools, or blood in the stool
* Weakness and fatigue
* Unintended weight loss

If you have symptoms, you should contact your health care provider and share your medical history and have a physical exam. Screening procedures include blood tests, biopsy (during a colonoscopy or sigmoidoscopy), and other imaging procedures (ACS, 2013).

Prostate Cancer

Although there is only limited data on the risk of prostate cancer (the most common type of cancer in men, among night-shift workers), one study in Japan revealed an association between rotating shift work and increased risk of prostate cancer (Bercz & Jaffe, 2012). Evidence suggests that this risk is due to the same factors as those outlined for breast cancer and colorectal cancers.

According to the ACS (2013), generally, early prostate cancers do not cause symptoms. More advanced prostate cancer symptoms might include a change in your urinary stream or blood in the urine. Sometimes, symptoms include pain in your back, hips, chest, or other areas. You might also experience numbness in the legs or feet. Early diagnosis is key and includes screening with a blood test for the prostate-specific antigen (PSA) and/or a digital rectal exam (DRE). More advanced prostate cancer may be diagnosed with a biopsy and various imaging procedures.

Stress and Depression

Nurses as a whole deal with multiple stressors while at work, but night-shift nurses experience additional stressors unique to the time of their shift. One of these stressors relates to the availability of help. Night shifts are often less well staffed compared to day shifts, meaning there are simply fewer people available to help with physically demanding tasks such as lifting or bathing patients. The staffing downturn also means there are fewer people to turn to for advice or psychological support when necessary. In addition, because the night shift is usually staffed by less senior nurses, not only are there fewer people, but often less-experienced people as compared to other shifts.

As if nurse staffing levels were not problematic enough, nurses are also subject to the stress of reduced staffing in other areas, such as pharmacy, laboratory, or supply. Night-shift nurses are often expected to run errands, draw blood, or mix intravenous medications in the absence of those disciplines, or wait longer for medications and supplies. The same can be said for medical staff support, where night-shift nurses often care for critically ill patients with minimal physician support. The push/pull between less staffing, more demands, and less-experienced staff can lead to high levels of anxiety and greater levels of job-related stress.

Not only do night-shift nurses suffer work-related stress, but also stress related to home life, social life, and sleep deprivation. While at work, the nurse's family and friends are comfortably sleeping. When the nurse arrives home, ready for sleep, everyone else is awakening and the day is just starting. Important engagements are missed, such as baseball games, parent-teacher conferences, family dinners, or even holidays, so that the nurse can sleep and be ready for her next shift.

These stressors, in conjunction with the circadian rhythm disruption and sleep deprivation often experienced by night-shift nurses, can also increase the risk of various health problems, including cardiovascular events. In addition, they can lead to unipolar depression, "a common psychological condition, consisting of feelings of low self-worth, sadness, lack of interest or pleasure in normally enjoyable activities, with an adverse effect on relationships and everyday functioning" (Wiebe, Cassoff, & Gruber, 2012).

 Compounding the problem is that depressed people are more prone to insomnia. In other words, the less sleep you get, the more likely you are to become depressed—and the more depressed you are, the less likely you are to fall asleep. A vicious cycle!

Two related theories have been proposed to explain the biological relationship between the sleep/wake system and depression. One of these theories relates to the prefrontal cortex (PFC), which is thought to play "a significant role in the coordination of sleep and wakefulness" (Wiebe et al., 2012) in addition to its involvement in mood regulation. Wiebe et al. explain: "The orbital and medial PFC are connected, either directly or indirectly, with the amygdala and hypothalamus structures in the limbic system, which are important for affect regulation. Sleep deprivation has been shown to lead to weaker functional connectivity between these areas, suggesting that impairment due to sleep problems affects mood regulation" (2012).

The other theory pertains to serotonin receptors. Serotonin is a neurotransmitter popularly thought to contribute to feelings of well-being and happiness. A recent study with sleep-deprived rats showed significant desensitization of serotonin receptors. "These findings suggest that sleep restriction leads to a decreased response to the presence of serotonin, thereby limiting the brain's ability to optimally use the serotonin available to it, and creating a situation that has also been found to be present for individuals suffering from unipolar depression" (Wiebe et al., 2012). A follow-up study revealed that receptor sensitivity was still not back to baseline levels even after seven days of recovery sleep.

A Word on Substance Abuse

According to Zee, "Research suggests a possible bidirectional association between sleep and substance abuse. Substance abuse may lead to sleep problems and sleep disturbances may be a risk factor for relapse in substance use" (2012). You might make the case, then, that this makes night-shift nurses at risk for substance abuse. Indeed, "Many shift workers turn to both prescription or over-the-counter drugs to help keep them awake and alert through the night" (Milano, n.d.). Smoking and alcohol consumption are also common among nurses to counteract stress. As a nurse on the night shift, you must take special care to ensure you avoid falling into this trap!

You can avoid the effects of depression by eating a healthy diet, exercising regularly, and maintaining close personal contacts. Seek out friends, join a professional group, find a hobby, develop a passion. Eat a balanced diet and move, move, move!

It is important to recognize the signs and symptoms of depression and to seek help if you believe you are depressed. If you feel tired, have no energy, cannot concentrate or focus, have difficulty remembering things, feel worthless or hopeless, feel irritable or restless, feel sad, or have lost interest in things you were previously interested in, you may be depressed. If you have thoughts of hurting yourself or have tried to hurt yourself, you should seek medical attention immediately.

Reproductive Issues

Women who work the night shift are more likely to be plagued with reproductive issues than their day-shift counterparts. Specifically, women who work the night shift are more likely to experience menstrual irregularities. In fact, "A study of 68 night-shift nurses of child-bearing age demonstrated that 53% of the women experienced changes in menstrual function, including changes in duration and flow of menses, as well as increased pain" (Bercz & Jaffe, 2012).

Moreover, working the night shift appears to affect women's fertility. One European study of 6,630 working women aged 25–44 years revealed that "rotating shift work was associated with a higher risk of subfecundity, which was defined as requiring more than 9.5 months of unprotected intercourse to achieve pregnancy" (Bercz & Jaffe, 2012). (Note that according to Bercz and Jaffe, "Having a male partner engaging in shift work did not impact fertility in this female population.")

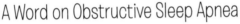

A Word on Obstructive Sleep Apnea

Some sleep deprivation may be due to obstructive sleep apnea (OSA). This is a condition that affects people regardless of the shift they work. Risk factors include "snoring and at least one of the following: obesity, depression, hypertentions, gastroesophageal reflux disease, congestive heart failure, large neck circumference, or a high Mallampati score" (Journal of Occupational and Environmental Medicine, 2011). A Mallampati score is related to the ease (low score) or difficulty (high score) of potential intubation. OSA is diagnosed by a sleep study. Treatment may include improving the sleep pattern and schedule, medications, use of oral appliances, or use of positive airway pressure (PAP) (Lerman et al., 2012).

General Tips for Healthy Living

As a nurse, you are in a unique position to serve as a role model for others—particularly with respect to health. Perhaps the American Nurses Association (n.d.) put it best:

A healthy nurse is a nurse who takes care of his or her personal health, safety, and wellness and lives life to their fullest capacity—physically, mentally, spiritually, and professionally. A healthy nurse is a better role model, educator, and advocate—personally, for the family, for the community, for the work environment, and for the patient. Nurses are 3.1 million strong and the most trusted profession, and have the power to make a difference! By choosing nutritious foods and an active lifestyle, managing stress, living tobacco-free, getting preventive immunizations and screenings, and choosing protective measures such as wearing sunscreen and bicycle helmets, nurses can set an example on how to BE healthy.

Following are just a few of the actions you can take to stay healthy and to promote health for others (Agency for Healthcare Research and Quality, 2010a; 2010b; Centers for Disease Control and Prevention, n.d.; Healthfinder.gov, n.d.a; n.d.b):

* **Get regular checkups.** If you don't have a chronic medical condition, see your health care provider at least once a year for a routine checkup and your dentist twice a year for routine dental cleaning and examinations.

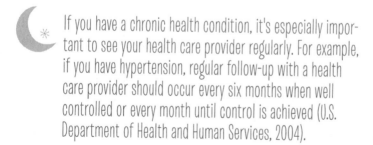

If you have a chronic health condition, it's especially important to see your health care provider regularly. For example, if you have hypertension, regular follow-up with a health care provider should occur every six months when well controlled or every month until control is achieved (U.S. Department of Health and Human Services, 2004).

* **Get the screenings you need, when you need them.** These might include screenings for breast, cervical, colorectal, and other forms of cancer; chlamydia, syphilis, or other sexually transmitted diseases; depression; diabetes; high blood pressure; high cholesterol; HIV; osteoporosis; and obesity.

Talk to your health care provider about which screenings are right for you and when you should have them.

* **Know and understand your numbers.** For a glimpse into your health status and risk for certain diseases, keep track of your blood pressure, blood sugar, cholesterol, BMI, and other numbers you may have.

* **Pay attention to signs and symptoms.** Are you experiencing excessive thirst? Have you noticed a strange rash or sore? Do you have shortness of breath? Be on the lookout for these and other signs and symptoms, and see your health care provider if they occur.

* **Take preventive medicines if you need them.** These might include aspirin (to prevent strokes) and vaccinations such as flu shots.

* **Maintain a healthy weight.** We have seen that being over-weight increases your risk of a whole host of health problems. Do not consume more calories than you burn.

* **Make healthy food choices.** Eat a variety of fruits, veg-etables, and whole grains each day and limit foods and drinks that are high in calories, sugar, salt, fat, and alcohol. In ad-dition to helping you to maintain a healthy weight, mak-ing good food choices can protect you from various health problems such as heart disease, type 2 diabetes, and even some forms of cancer. (For more on healthy food choices, see Chapter 4.)

* **Be physically active.** Regular exercise increases the likeli-hood that you'll live a longer, healthier life. Performing activ-ities for at least 2.5 hours per week that raise your breathing and heart rates and strengthen your muscles will help you to maintain weight; reduce high blood pressure; reduce your risk for type 2 diabetes, heart attack, stroke, and several forms of cancer; reduce arthritis pain and associated disability; reduce the risk for osteoporosis and falls; and reduce symptoms of depression and anxiety. (For more on exercise, see Chapter 5.)

* **Manage stress.** Balance work, home, and play. Seek support from family and friends. Stay positive. Take time to relax and get adequate sleep. If needed, get help or counseling.

* **Limit alcohol intake.** Avoid drinking more than one alcoholic beverage per day.

* **Don't smoke or use other forms of tobacco.** Quitting smoking can greatly decrease cardiovascular risk, not to mention the likelihood you'll contract various forms of cancer and other diseases.

Tips on Quitting Smoking

Of course, talking about quitting smoking is the easy part. Actually doing it takes commitment and willpower. Before you quit smoking, write five or ten reasons to quit. Reasons should be tangible and measureable, such as "I want to save $10 a day by quitting smoking," to immeasurable but compelling, such as "I want to enjoy my grandchildren." Post these reasons with other visual cues, such as pictures, in a conspicuous place.

While trying to quit smoking, identify and avoid triggers for smoking, such as drinking alcohol. Substitute other behaviors, such as exercising, doing crafts, or reading, to avoid caving in to cravings. Finally, enlist the help of addiction specialists or even pharmacologic means if necessary. Many organizations, such as the American Lung Association, the American Heart Association, and the American Cancer Society, offer support and assistance to people who wish to quit smoking. Search the Internet for tips and resources and decide to quit smoking today.

References

American Cancer Society (ACS). (2013). The American Cancer Society / Information and resources for cancer: Breast, colon, lung, prostate, skin. Retrieved from www.cancer.org/index

American Diabetes Association. (2002). Screening for diabetes. *Diabetes Care, 25*(1), S21-23. Retrieved from http://care.diabetesjournals.org/content/25/suppl_1/s21.full#T2

American Nurses Association (ANA). (n.d.). Healthy nurse. *Nursing World*. Retrieved from http://www.nursingworld.org/MainMenuCategories/WorkplaceSafety/Healthy-Nurse

Arble, D. M., Bass, J., Laposky, A. D., Vitaterna, M. H., & Turek, F. W. (2009). Circadian timing of food intake contributes to weight gain. *Obesity, 17*(11), 2100-2102. Retrieved from http://onlinelibrary.wiley.com/doi/10.1038/oby.2009.264/full

Bercz, P. A., & Jaffe, F. (2012). Adverse health effects of shift work and shift work sleep disorder. *Dialogue and Diagnosis, 2*(1), 13-20. Retrieved from http://www.osteopathic.org/inside-aoa/news-and-publications/Documents/dd-13-20-bercz-jaffe-march-2012.pdf

Bogglid, H., & Knutsson, A. (1999). Shift work, risk factors and cardiovascular disease. *Scandanavian Journal of Work, Environment and Health, 25*(2), 85-99. Retrieved from http://www.jstor.org/discover/10.2307/40966872?uid=3739664&uid=2&uid=4&uid=3739256&sid=21101788080121

Bumgardner, W. (2008). Walking reduces breast cancer risk. *About.com*. Retrieved from http://about.com/cs/cancerprevention/a/bcnursestudy.htm

Eberly, R., & Feldman, H. (2010). Obesity and shift work in the general population. *The Internet Journal of Allied Health Sciences and Practice, 8*(3). Retrieved from http://ijahsp.nova.edu/articles/Vol8Num3/pdf/feldman.pdf

Esquirol, Y., Perret, B., Ruidavets, J. B., Marquie, J. C., Dienne, E., Niezborala, M., & Ferrieres, J. (2011). Shift work and cardiovascular risk factors: New knowledge from the past decade. *Archives of Cardiovascular Disease, 104*, 636-668.

Gordon, S. (2011). Rotating shift work may boost women's diabetes risk. *U.S. News and World Report*. Retrieved from http://health.usnews.com/health-news/diet-fitness/diabetes/articles/2011/12/06/rotating-shift-work-may-boost-womens-diabetes-risk

Grundy, S. M., Brewer, H. B., Cleeman, J. I., Smith, S. C., Jr., & Lenfant, C. (2004). Definition of metabolic syndrome: Report of the National Heart, Lung, and Blood Institute/American Heart Association Conference on Scientific Issues Related to Definition. *Circulation, 109*, 433-38.

Healthfinder.gov. (n.d.a). Eat healthy. Retrieved from http://www.healthfinder.gov/HealthTopics/Category/nutrition-and-physical-activity/nutrition

Healthfinder.gov. (n.d.b). Get active. Retrieved from http://www.healthfinder.gov/HealthTopics/Category/nutrition-and-physical-activity/physical-activity

Journal of Occupational and Environmental Medicine. (2011). Shift work and sleep: Optimizing health, safety , and performance. *Journal of Occupational and Environmental Medicine, 53*(5), 1–10. [supplemental material].

Kawachi, I., Colditz, G. A., Stamfer, M. J., Willett, W. C., Manson, J. E., Speizer, F. E., & Hennekins, C. H. (1995). Prospective study of shift work and risk of coronary artery disease in women. *Circulation, 92*, 3178-3182. Retrieved from http://circ.ahajournals.org/content/92/11/3178.full

Lerman, S. E., Eskin, E., Flower, D., George, E., Gerson, B., Hartenbaum, M., ...Moore-Ede, M. (2012). Fatigue risk management in the workplace. *Journal of Occupational and Environmental Medicine, 54*(2), 231-258.

Lieu, S. J., Curhan, G. C., Schernhammer, E. S., & Forman, J. P. (2011). Rotating night shift work and disparate hypertension risk in African-Americans. *Journal of Hypertension, 30*(1), 61-66.

Mann, D. (2012). Heart attack, stroke more common in shift workers. *WebMD*. Retrieved from http://www.webmd.com/heart-disease/news/20120726/heart-attack-stroke-more-common-in-shift-workers

McSweeney, J. C., Cody, M., & Crane, P. B. (2001). Do you know them when you see them? Women's prodromal and acute symptoms of myocardial infarction. *Journal of Cardiovascular Nursing, 15*(3), 2619-2623.

McSweeney, J. C., Cody, M., O'Sullivan, P., Elberson, K., Moser, D. K., & Garvin, B. J. (2003). Women's early warning symptoms of acute myocardial infarction. *Circulation, 108*(21), 2619-23.

Milano, C. (n.d.). Night workers face array of difficulties. Retrieved from http://www.carolmilano.com/nightshift.html

Pan, A., Schernhammer, E. S., Sun, Q., & Hu, F. B. (2011). Rotating night shift work and risk of type 2 diabetes: Two prospective cohort studies in women. *PLOS Medicine*. Retrieved from http://www.plosmedicine.org/article/info%3Adoi%2F10.1371%2Fjournal.pmed.1001141

Persson, M., & Martensson, J. (2006). Situations influencing habits in diet and exercise among nurses working night shift. *Journal of Nursing Management, 14*(5), 414-423.

Rogers, A. (2008). The effects of fatigue and sleepiness on nurse performance and patient safety. In R. G. Hughes (Ed.), *Patient safety and quality: An evidence-based handbook for nurses.* (AHRQ Publication No. 08-0043). Retrieved from http://www.ncbi.nlm.nih.gov/pubmed/21328747

Schernhammer, E. S., Laden, F., Speizer, F. E., Willett, W. C., Hunter, D. J., Kawachi, I.,...Colditz, G. A. (2003). Night-shift work and risk of colorectal cancer in the Nurses' Health Study. *Journal of the National Cancer Institute, 95*(11), 825-828.

Shochat, T. (2012). Impact of lifestyle and technology developments on sleep. *Nature and Science of Sleep, 2012*(4), 19-31. Retrieved from http://www.dovepress.com/impact-of-lifestyle-and-technology-developments-on-sleep-peer-reviewed-article-NSS

Stevens, R. G. (2009). Light-at-night, circadian disruption and breast cancer: Assessment of existing evidence. *International Journal of Epidemiology, 38*(4), 963–970. Retrieved from http://www.ncbi.nlm.nih.gov/pmc/articles/PMC2734067/

Stokowski, L. (2012, January 24). Help me make it through the night (shift). *Medscape Today*. Retrieved from http://www.medscape.com/viewarticle/757050

U.S. Department of Health and Human Services, Agency for Healthcare Research and Quality. (2010a). Men: Stay healthy at any age. Retrieved from http://www.ahrq.gov/patients-consumers/patient-involvement/healthy-men/healthy-men.html

U.S. Department of Health and Human Services, Agency for Healthcare Research and Quality. (2010b). Women: Stay healthy at any age. Retrieved from http://www.ahrq.gov/legacy/ppip/healthywom.htm

U.S. Department of Health and Human Services, Centers for Disease Control and Prevention. (n.d.). Tips for a safe and healthy life. Retrieved from http://www.cdc.gov/family/tipsgen.pdf

U.S. Department of Health and Human Services, National Institutes of Health, National Heart, Lung and Blood Institute. (2004). The seventh report of the Joint National Committee on Prevention, Detection, Evaluation, and Treatment of High Blood Pressure. NIH Publication No. 04-5230.

Vyas, M., Garg, A., Iansavichus, A., Costella, J., Donner, A., Laugsand, L....Hackman, D. (2012). Shift work and vascular events: Systemic review and meta-analysis. *British Medical Journal, 345*:e4800.

Wiebe, S. T., Cassoff, J., & Gruber, R. (2012). Sleep patterns and the risk for unipolar depression: A review. *Nature and Science of Sleep, 2012*(4), 63-71. Retrieved from http://www.dovepress.com/sleep-patterns-and-the-risk-for-unipolar-depression-a-review-peer-reviewed-article-NSS

Zee, P. (2012). Struggling with shift work disorder. *Medscape Education*. Retrieved from http://www.medscape.org/viewarticle/769403_12

4

Those who think they have no time for healthy eating will sooner or later have to find time for illness.

-Edward Stanley

Healthful Eating

IN THIS CHAPTER

Making healthful food selections

Ideas for eating well at work

Combating GI issues

Most people know that healthful eating is important. What we eat is one of the key determinants of good health (Harvard School of Public Health, n.d.). Sadly, many Americans have very poor eating habits. Sweets, desserts, sodas, and alcoholic drinks account for nearly 25% of all calories the average American consumes. In contrast, fruits and vegetables comprise a mere 10% of Americans' caloric intake (CBS News, 2010). Moreover, Americans are consuming more calories than they did 30 years ago—roughly 570 calories more per day (Moisse, 2011). The result? An increasingly overweight (even obese) and unhealthy population.

Unfortunately, these problems appear to be particularly prevalent among night-shift workers. In one study of 27 night-shift nurses, many reported "eating foods high in sugar in order to override the feeling of tiredness" (Eberly & Feldman, 2010). Moreover, "Sweet foods and junk food were readily consumed due to ease of access compared to an alternatively healthy snack" (Eberly & Feldman, 2010). According to Eberly and Feldman, these findings have been replicated in other small studies, as have the preference among night-shift workers for cold and fast food, and tendencies among night-shift workers to "nibble rather than have a meal" and eat fewer well-balanced meals. These studies do not explicitly define a relationship between these behaviors and the higher incidence of obesity among night-shift workers. However, some relationship is likely.

 As mentioned in Chapter 3, "Health Issues and Prevention," matters for night-shift workers are complicated by the circadian rhythm, which regulates, among other things, digestive functions. As a result, food eaten may not be "in synch" with digestion.

Making Healthful Food Selections

So what's a night-shift nurse to do? Unfortunately, there's a lot of confusing—and conflicting—information about proper nutrition. The answer to the question "What should I eat?" is quite simple (Harvard School of Public Health, n.d.):

> Eat a plant-based diet rich in fruits, vegetables, and whole grains; choose foods with healthful fats, such as olive and canola oil, nuts and fatty fish; limit red meat and foods that are high in saturated fat; and avoid foods that contain trans fats. Drink water and other healthful beverages, and limit sugary drinks and salt. Most important of all is keeping calories in check, so you can avoid weight gain, which makes exercise a key partner to a healthful diet.

It's also important to think about how much of each food you should eat. An excellent guide is the Choose My Plate paradigm (ChooseMyPlate.gov, n.d.). It indicates that half of your plate (at each meal!) should be filled with fruits and vegetables (with an emphasis on vegetables), one quarter with lean protein, and one quarter with whole grain or complex carbohydrate foods such as brown rice, whole wheat bread, or half of a baked sweet potato. Add a small serving of low-fat or fat-free dairy products to provide calcium and protein.

Here are a few more good eating tips to keep in mind (ChooseMyPlate. gov, n.d., Harvard School of Public Health, n.d.):

* Balance calories. Eat only the number of calories that you need for a day.

* Eat a diet rich in whole grains, vegetables, and fruits to increase fiber intake.

* Choose fruits and vegetables with bright colors—red peppers, strawberries, oranges, carrots, peaches, winter squash, etc.

* Make at least half, preferably more, of your grains whole grains.

* Choose food with healthful fats, such as plant oils, nuts, and fish. Avoid foods that are high in saturated fat or that contain trans fat.

* Choose fish, poultry, nuts, and beans rather than red meat.

* Choose fresh or minimally processed foods whenever possible.
* Choose low-sodium versions of foods (check the labels).

 Just because you're trying to eat healthfully doesn't mean you have to give up all your favorite foods. Consult a registered dietitian or chef to help "decalorize" your favorite recipes!

* Use lower-fat salad dressings, such as vinaigrettes. Skip the croutons and cheese, and limit the nuts due to their high calorie content.
* Drink water (best for quenching thirst) or unsweetened beverages.
* Go easy on milk and juice.
* Limit alcohol intake.
* Avoid foods that are high in salt, saturated fat, and sugar, such as cakes, cookies, ice cream, candy, hot dogs, fried chicken, most soups, ribs, bacon, and sausage. Save these foods for an occasional treat or a special occasion.
* Avoid fried foods. Foods that are fried (or that are too spicy) may cause indigestion or heartburn.
* Use small cups and plates to limit portion size. Measuring your food can also be helpful.
* Enjoy your food and eat less, paying attention to hunger and fullness cues.

 Eat a snack and make a list before you go to the grocery store. This will help you avoid impulse buys, which are almost always less healthful. Remember that the healthiest foods are found around the perimeter of the grocery store, and the least healthful ones are everywhere else!

Simple Meal and Snack Ideas

Here are a few ideas for healthful meals and snacks:

*   Turkey sandwich on whole-grain bread with a green salad or fruit on the side. Try hummus on the bread instead of mayonnaise and substitute spinach for iceberg lettuce.

*   Two tablespoons peanut butter and four or five thin banana slices on two slices of whole-grain bread. Finish the meal with one medium apple.

*   One half of a whole-wheat pita bread filled with two ounces sliced turkey, one ounce Swiss cheese, cucumber slices, and spinach leaves with a small amount of plain Greek yogurt (instead of mayonnaise).

*   Two-egg (or two-egg-white) omelet with two slices unprocessed low-fat cheese and your choice of veggies, plus two slices whole-grain toast, spread with one teaspoon of peanut butter.

*   Salad made of quinoa (a grain-like product that's high in protein), chopped vegetables, and kidney or garbanzo beans, dressed with a teaspoon of olive oil and a teaspoon of balsamic vinegar.

*   One half cup of Greek yogurt mixed with one half cup of unsweetened whole-grain cereal that contains at least 5 grams of fiber per serving.

*   Two pieces of low-fat string cheese, 10 unsalted pretzels, and one banana.

*   One-quarter cup mixed almonds and pistachio nuts with one-quarter cup dried cranberries or raisins and a low-sugar beverage.

*   One hard-boiled egg (or two hard-boiled egg whites), eight small whole-grain crackers, and 20 grapes.

Ideas for Eating Well at Work

Of course, the trick is to adhere to these principles—something that's especially difficult when you hit that 4 a.m. lull. It's also true that "food service on the night shift is often limited to a few choices in the hospital cafeteria or as a last resort, what is available in the vending machine" (Eberly & Feldman, 2010)! The following list highlights actions you can take to maximize your ability to feel better on and off shift duty (EatRight Ontario, n.d.; MedicineNet.com, 2006; Noelcke, n.d.; Wong, 2012; Working Nights, 2009):

* **Bring food from home.** That way, you won't have to consume empty calories from vending-machine snacks or resort to eating fast food. Bringing food from home involves planning in advance so that you have nutritious, packable, tasty foods in your refrigerator, freezer, and cupboard. Consider packing your meal and snacks for your next shift before you fall asleep after the last one to make it easy to "grab and go" as you head back out for work.

 Consider planning one or two less healthful meals each week to give yourself a break. This may also give you more fortitude to resist less healthful foods brought in by colleagues or patients' families. "Relaxing your diet one day every week so that you can eat some of your favorite unhealthful foods will actually benefit you, by stimulating the body to release more of the hormone leptin, which increases your metabolism" (Samuels, 2011).

* **Gear up.** Invest in appropriate containers (available at all price points) and a lunch bag you like, preferably with a freezable ice pack included.

On your day off, try making a large batch of bean-rich chili, low-fat lasagna, or low-fat cheese enchiladas. Freeze it in meal-sized portions. Then grab a portion on the way out the door before your next shift.

* **Avoid the vending machine.** If you must use a vending machine, check for a "healthy food" symbol that identifies items lower in fat, sodium, sugar, and calories. Choose a small bag of peanuts, a whole-grain bar, peanut-butter crackers, or whole-grain crackers or chips.

* **Avoid the all-night cafeteria and don't order take-out.** If you must order take-out or choose from the all-night cafeteria menu, make healthful choices. Pick small sandwiches on multigrain bread, wraps made with grilled vegetables and low-fat cheese, or chicken or minestrone soup with multigrain bread on the side.

FROM THE TRENCHES

Our cafeteria is open for night-shift nurses from 11 p.m. to 2:30 a.m. each day. The color coding of healthier choices was initiated by our food and nutrition department to assist employees and anyone using the cafeteria to make healthier choices. We now have three colors: Green is best, with low saturated fat; yellow is caution, with less than 7.5 g saturated fat; and red is poor, with greater than 7.5 grams saturated fat.

–Barbara Brunt, MA, MN, RN-BC, NE-BC

* **Don't use food as entertainment.** Night-shift workers often snack out of boredom or to stay awake. You'll gain weight if you eat to pass the time.

* **Be mindful.** Take a few moments before eating to take some deep breaths and pay attention to the way your body feels. When you begin to eat, savor the bites and don't rush. This will help you avoid overeating.

* **Do not skip meals.** Be prepared for those days when you can't eat a "real meal" during your shift because of the pace of the shift. Always keep a high-protein meal supplement bar, a bottle of water, a piece of fruit, and small packet of nuts or a whole-grain cereal bar in your backpack or purse.

* **Time your main meal.** If you start work in the afternoon, have your main meal in the middle of the day rather than in the middle of your shift. If you're working nights, eat your main meal before your shift starts, preferably between 5 and 7 p.m.

* **Eat small portions throughout your shift.** Eat small, regular meals. As noted by Wong (2012), "Eating small portions throughout your shift will help your body maintain a regular sugar level and will also keep you feeling energized."

 Eat at least 150-200 calories (40-50 of them from protein) every four hours to keep your blood sugar and energy levels stable.

* **Fuel up on complex carbs.** Choose carbohydrates that are low in fat and high in fiber, such as pasta, grains, whole-grain bread, and vegetables. These release energy slowly over a long period of time, in contrast to foods high in sugar, such as candy bars, which can cause a sugar high followed by a crash.

* **Eat protein foods.** Protein foods increase alertness and give your muscles the building blocks to make good use of the exercise you get throughout your shift.

* **Have a late-night pickup.** When you start to feel tired, a snack with a little protein provides sustained energy. This can help keep you alert when your body is programmed for sleep.

* **Don't eat a huge meal at the end of your shift.** For some people, this habit can cause stomach upset and disrupted slumber. Do eat a light snack of low-fat yogurt, fruit, or whole-grain toast before you sleep.

* **Consume some caffeine before or early in your shift.** Caffeine, found in beverages such as coffee and cola as well as in chocolate, stimulates the central nervous system and provides an energy boost. Experts recommend a maximum of 200–300 milligrams daily. Stop caffeine consumption several hours before your shift ends to ensure it does not interfere with your ability to sleep. Caffeine's effects may linger for six to eight hours, or longer.

* **Drink lots of water.** Keep a water bottle close by and drink regularly throughout your shift. This prevents dehydration, which can make you tired and cause cramps and headaches. By the time you are thirsty, dehydration has likely already set in. Cut back a bit on your fluid intake during the last few hours of your shift or your sleep may be interrupted by bathroom breaks.

* **Stay active during your shift.** Some light exercise midway through your shift will increase your energy, improve your mood, and help you sleep better. If you have an extra break, do some stretches or go for a brisk walk. If possible, always use a restroom that is the furthest from your work station.

FROM THE TRENCHES

Eat right. Hydrate often. If you are uncertain about times, use this guide: Your breakfast is your family's dinner, lunch is at work, and dinner is your family's breakfast. That way, you only have to think about changing one meal on your days off. For energy, eat lots of fruits, veggies, nuts, yogurt, and hard-boiled eggs. This menu does a body good with all of the potlucks and celebrations the night shift has time to offer. Drink fluids throughout your shift but only lightly before sleep to prevent the urges from waking you.

–Kathy Alkire, BSN, RN

Healthcare organizations can help motivate employees to eat healthfully. One hospital has nightly tea time for its nurses. This was started by the nurses as a way of developing community and also to make sure they were taking care of themselves by taking a break and eating. Another hospital sponsors a monthly night-shift meal, for which a chef comes in to prepare the meal and to show night-shift workers more healthful options.

Combating GI Issues

Even more than the average American, some 50% of permanent night-shift workers grapple with appetite disturbances or gastrointestinal problems (Bercz & Jaffe, 2012). These include the following:

* Abdominal pain
* Constipation
* Diarrhea
* Heartburn
* Indigestion
* Loss of appetite
* Nausea

If shift work seems to make you constipated, fluid, fiber, and activity will help. Look for snack foods (such as cereals, nutrition bars, dried plums, and so on) that contain 5-10 grams of fiber per serving and meal options (such as lentil soup, black-bean burritos, or brown rice and vegetables) made with high-fiber foods. Each time you eat a high-fiber item, drink 8-10 ounces of water or a low-calorie, hot beverage such as herbal tea. Keep moving whenever you can.

Researchers have noted a threefold increased prevalence of colon polyps, stomach ulcers, and ulcerative colitis among night-shift workers. (Bercz & Jaffe, 2012). Gastrointestinal disturbances include the following:

* **Peptic ulcers.** According to Bercz and Jaffe, "Several large-scale studies have demonstrated statistically significant increases in the risk of gastric and duodenal ulcers in night-shift and rotating-shift workers compared to day workers" (2012). Indeed, some researchers suggest the risk of peptic ulcer disease among night-shift workers is twice that in daytime workers (Sugisawa & Uehata, 1998).

* **Gastroesophageal reflux disease (GERD).** Researchers in China have observed that night-shift work is associated with GERD, even when adjustments are made for such factors as age, work burden, marital status, and eating habits (Li, Y.M., Du, J., Zhang, H., & Yu, C.H., 2008).

* **Inflammatory bowel disease (IBD).** IBD—particularly ulcerative colitis and Crohn's disease—is exacerbated by disruptions in sleep, which are common among night-shift workers (Bercz & Jaffe, 2012).

* **Irritable bowel syndrome (IBS).** IBS, characterized by chronic bouts of abdominal pain, bloating, and alteration of bowel habits (i.e., alternating constipation and diarrhea), is the most common functional bowel disorder. A 2010 study showed that "participation in shift work, especially rotating shift work, was associated with the development of IBS and abdominal pain—independent of sleep quality" (Bercz & Jaffe, 2012).

Unfortunately, there are no nutritional means by which to prevent ulcers or IBD. For its part, IBS is associated in some people with intake of certain types of foods, such as those rich in FODMAPs. (FODMAPs include fructans, as in wheat, rye, garlic, artichokes, asparagus, and chocolate; galactans, as in legumes and beans; fructose, found in many fruits; and polyols, found in some fruit as well as in artificial sweeteners. These are poorly absorbed in the small intestine.)

However, it's more closely associated with personality types and work schedules. GERD can be managed by avoiding foods like peppermint that relax the lower esophageal sphincter (LES).

There are some ways to reduce your risk for GI problems, including the following:

* Pace your eating. Don't eat too quickly!
* Eat moderate portions. Don't overeat.
* Select foods that are low in fat and high in fiber.
* Watch your caffeine intake. Reduce or eliminate caffeine as needed.
* Stay hydrated!
* Increase your physical activity
* Maintain a healthful weight or lose weight if needed.

FROM THE TRENCHES

Our staff, mostly night shift, participated in a weight-loss and weight-gain challenge from April 2012 to June 2012. The challenge was to see who could lose the most percentage of body weight in eight weeks. On the flip side, to make it an equal opportunity for all, we also had a weight-gain challenge (for those who needed to gain weight). It was a fun challenge. All weights were taken and stored in a confidential place. All staff who participated were winners in the end.

–Tiare Geolina Gonzales, MBA, BSN, RN, CCRN

References

Bercz, P. A., & Jaffe, F. (2012). Adverse health effects of shift work and shift work sleep disorder. *Dialogue and Diagnosis, 2*(1), 13-20. Retrieved from http://www.osteopathic.org/inside-aoa/news-and-publications/Documents/dd-13-20-bercz-jaffe-march-2012.pdf

CBS News. (2010). How Americans eat today. Retrieved from http://www.cbsnews.com/2100-500165_162-6086647.html

ChooseMyPlate.gov. (n.d.). Food groups. Retrieved from http://www.choosemyplate.gov/food-groups/

EatRight Ontario. (n.d.). Nutrition tips for shift workers. Retrieved from https://www.eatrightontario.ca/en/Articles/Workplace-wellness/Nutrition-Tips-for-Shift-Workers

Eberly, R., & Feldman, H. (2010). Obesity and shift work in the general population. *The Internet Journal of Allied Health Sciences and Practice, 8*(3). Retrieved from http://ijahsp.nova.edu/articles/Vol8Num3/pdf/feldman.pdf

Harvard School of Public Health. (n.d.). The nutrition source. Retrieved from http://www.hsph.harvard.edu/nutritionsource/

Li, Y. M., Du, J., Zhang, H., & Yu, C. H. (2008). Epidemiological investigation in outpatients with symptomatic gastroesophageal reflux from the department of medicine in Zhejiang Province, East China. *Journal Gastroenterology and Hepatology, 23*(2), 283-289.

MedicineNet.com. (2006). A hard day's night for Weight Watchers on the night shift. Retrieved from http://www.medicinenet.com/script/main/art.asp?articlekey=77354

Moisse, K. (2011, June 28). The American diet then and now: How snacking is expanding the country's waistline. *ABC News.* Retrieved from http://abcnews.go.com/Health/w_DietAndFitness/american-diet-now-snacking-expanding-countrys-waistline/story?id=13948594

Noelcke, L. (n.d.). How to work the third shift and stay healthy. *SparkPeople.* Retrieved from http://www.sparkpeople.com/resource/wellness_articles.asp?id=217

Samuels, M. (2011). Healthy eating habits for people who work nights. *Livestrong.* Retrieved from www.livestrong.com/article/371078-healthy-eating-heabits-for-people-who-work-nights

Sugisawa, A., & Uehata, T. (1998). Onset of peptic ulcer and its relation to work-related factors and life events: A prospective study. *Journal of Occupational Health, 40*(1), 22-31.

Wong, M. (2012). 9 survival tips for night shift nurses. *healthecareers Network.* Retrieved from http://www.healthecareers.com/article/9-survival-tips-for-night-shift-nurses/169114

Working Nights. (2009). Be careful when and what you eat, when working night shift. Retrieved from http://www.workingnights.com/blog/2009/09/17/be-careful-when-you-eat-when-working-shift-work-no-greasy-fries-and-burgers-anymore/

5

Lack of activity destroys the good condition of every human being, while movement and methodical physical exercise save it and preserve it.

–Plato

Exercise Benefits

IN THIS CHAPTER

The benefits of exercise

Exercise options

Getting started

Exercising at work

Night-shift nurses spend their work lives caring for others—often at the expense of their own health. Many blogs, surveys, and websites delve into the reasons why night-shift nurses ignore their own health in this manner. Some of the explanations include:

* "[The] night shift is fatiguing even if you get 6-8 hours of sleep."
* "On my days off, all I want to do is sleep and eat."
* "I am awake all night and then awake all day with my baby."

Although there are many reasons for not exercising, we know there are many benefits to including exercise each day or night! Indeed, exercise can go a long way toward helping night-shift nurses maintain their health and, in particular, their energy levels. As noted by Eberly and Feldman (2010) of night-shift workers:

> Lack of energy to engage in physical activity [is] a major contributor to weight gain in those who work during the night. Unfortunately, this can be a vicious cycle difficult to break if not addressed quickly. Exercise energizes the body. Clearly, individuals who do not exercise do not benefit from the energy provided, and therefore continue in their feeling of lassitude.

In addition to helping night-shift workers maintain their energy levels, exercise can play a part in obtaining higher-quality sleep. Indeed, it "might even be the key to a good day's rest" (Eberly & Feldman, 2010). And because night-shift work is often physically taxing, building strength through exercise can be critical for the night-shift nurse's stamina.

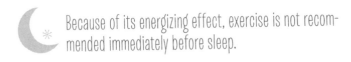
Because of its energizing effect, exercise is not recommended immediately before sleep.

The Benefits of Exercise

Regardless of whether you work the night shift or a regular day schedule, exercising offers countless health benefits. Here are just a few important benefits of exercise:

* **Weight loss.** According to the American College of Sports Medicine (ACSM; 2009, 2010), everyone should ideally perform light to moderate (40–60% of your maximum heart rate) exercise for 60–90 minutes, seven days a week, in order to lose weight. This could be, for example, walking, running, biking, swimming, or aerobic classes. Resistance training should be used as an adjunct to the aerobic exercise. (Roitman & LaFontaine, 2012). If your goal is simply to maintain your weight, the consensus is that you need to exercise for 30 minutes, "most days of the week" (Roitman & LaFontaine, 2012).

 For most people, diet and exercise combined will prove to be the most effective method for losing weight.

* **Improvement of stress levels.** When people are stressed, they experience an increase in cortisol, a hormone released from the adrenal gland in response to stress. The main function of cortisol is to prepare for "fight or flight." Cortisol has an immunosuppressive effect, meaning that bodies having continuously high levels of cortisol experience an increased risk of illness or infection (Mahoney, 2011). Regular exercise, however, minimizes the release of cortisol (Mahoney, 2011).

* **Reduction in coronary artery disease (CAD).** A study by Yusuf et al., the INTERHEART study, concluded that regular exercise (in addition to other modifiable risk factors) reduces the incidence of myocardial infarction (MI) by more than 75% (2004).

* **Management of diabetes.** A four-year study by Knowler et al. has shown that exercise and weight loss were more effective in controlling type 2 diabetes than the diabetes medication metformin (2002).

* **Management of blood pressure.** Regular exercise has shown a decrease of 5–7 mmHg within a four-week period of both systolic blood pressure (SBP) and diastolic blood pressure (DBP) for those with documented hypertension (Roitman & LaFontaine, 2012).

* **Enhanced sleep.** According to the National Sleep Foundation, 74% of adults in the U.S. have problems sleeping. Scientists have shown that regular exercisers spend more time in slow-wave sleep. This is a period of non–rapid eye movement (NREM) sleep during which a person's sleep, brain activity, respiration, blood pressure, heart rate, metabolism, and body temperature slow down. The result? A deep, restful state (Nieman, 2005). Better sleep, enhanced by exercise, will help you to awaken feeling well rested.

* **Reduction in the incidence of some cancers.** Researchers have shown that exercise can contribute to a reduction in breast cancer, colon cancer, and possibly lung and endometrial cancers. According to the ACSM (2010), physical activity involves several mechanisms that may influence cancer risks: improved circulation, ventilation, immune surveillance, and reduced free-radical buffering.

* **Prevention of osteoporosis (loss of bone).** The Cleveland Clinic and Mayo Clinic recommend weight-bearing exercise as one of the primary ways to build bone density, which helps stave off osteoporosis (Porter, 2010).

* **Improvement of muscle and heart-lung fitness.** The ACSM (2010) recommends a minimum of 20 minutes per day, 4 to 5 days per week, to improve cardiorespiratory fitness.

* **Decreased falls.** Physical activity, including muscle-strengthening activities, can help in reducing your risk of falling (Centers for Disease Control and Prevention, 2011).

* **Lower risk of depression.** As mentioned in Chapter 3, "Health Issues and Prevention," night-shift nurses are subject to a great number of stressors, both at work and at home. These stressors, along with the circadian rhythm disruption and sleep deprivation often experienced by night-shift nurses,

can lead to various health problems, including unipolar depression. Fortunately, according to Mayo Clinic, exercise can help ease the symptoms of depression: "The links between anxiety, depression and exercise aren't entirely clear—but working out can definitely help you relax and make you feel better. Exercise may also help keep anxiety and depression from coming back once you're feeling better" (Mayo Clinic, 2011).

In addition to the benefits just mentioned, there are several short-term, temporary, or *subacute*, benefits to exercise. These are "benefits that occur immediately following, and because of, each exercise session. They are different from the acute benefits, such as heart rate, blood pressure, and other physiological changes" (da Nobrega, 2005). Some examples of subacute benefits include the following:

* Decrease in triglycerides
* Increase in high-density lipoproteins (higher intensity exercise may be required)
* Decrease in low-density lipoproteins (higher intensity exercise may be required)
* Decrease in cholesterol
* Decrease in inflammation (low to moderate intensity exercise may be required)
* Increase in glucose metabolism (longer duration, lower intensity exercise may be required)

In short, exercise improves your chances of living longer…and living healthier!

Exercise Options

For many, the word "exercise" calls to mind such repetitive activities as running laps or performing sit-ups. But the fact is, any physical activity—be it the more traditional running, lifting weights, playing basketball, swimming, cycling, or doing other popular fitness activities, or less strenuous activities such as gardening, washing your car, or taking a stroll around the block—can help you achieve your fitness goals (Mayo Clinic, 2011).

 Of course, you should check with your health care provider before embarking on any new exercise routine, particularly if you have any preexisting medical conditions.

FROM THE TRENCHES

Just as "day" people exercise before work, so should you by going to the gym, working out to a video, or maintaining a routine on your exercise equipment. Walk at break time (my colleagues and I did lunges down the halls for months until we realized that there was a security camera!). Enjoy a nice swim, walk, or bike ride in the cool of the morning after work.

–Kathy Alkire, BSN, RN

Perhaps even more important is the realization that exercise need not be miserable. In fact, it can be downright fun! Take, for example, walking, which is inexpensive and does not require any special equipment (except a good pair of walking shoes). Walking, particularly with friends, is a fun, safe, and effective way to reduce stress, lose weight, reduce blood pressure, decrease serum cholesterol, and increase HDL levels. The Nurses' Health Study has demonstrated that nurses who walked three hours per week had a 34% reduction in their risk of stroke (Hu et al., 2000) and that nurses who walked quickly at least three hours a week reduced their risk of coronary artery disease by 35% (Manson et al., 1999). Walking has even been shown to reduce the risk of certain types of cancer and is thought to help the body adapt to the disruption in circadian rhythm related to night-shift work. This is particularly true if walking at a brisk pace—between 3 and 3.9 miles per hour (Bumgardner, 2008). In addition to walking, don't forget about hiking. Hiking up and down hills adds to the difficulty. Hiking also gives the added benefit of enabling you to commune with nature, which can do wonders for your mood.

Decrease the effects of social isolation, call a friend, and take a walk! Wondering where to walk? Use the American Heart Association's My Heart My Life Walking Paths app. Find it online: www.startwalkingnow.org/WalkingPathApp.jsp.

Here are a few more examples of exercise options that you might enjoy:

* **Kayaking.** Many parks enable visitors to rent kayaks. If you're a beginner, consider joining a kayaking group. It is amazing the "burn" you will feel after just 30 minutes to one hour of kayaking.

* **Tennis.** For a 150-pound person, playing 30 minutes of tennis burns approximately 285 calories. As an added bonus, it can be a highly social activity!

* **Golfing.** Playing nine holes of golf while towing your clubs (rather than riding in a cart) is great exercise. After all, you're essentially taking a two-hour walk!

* **Horseback riding.** Horseback riding is a great way to work muscles throughout your body—the shoulders and back, arms and hands, abdominals, thighs, and calves.

* **Water skiing.** Water skiing, which burns roughly 395 calories per hour, promotes considerable upper and lower body strength, muscular endurance, and good balance. Once you have mastered basic skiing, you can challenge yourself to slalom or trick skiing!

* **Ice skating.** Ice skating at a relatively slow speed (less than 9 miles per hour) burns 325 calories per hour for individuals weighing 130 pounds. Pick up the pace to burn even more calories!

* **Snow skiing and snowboarding.** If you live near a ski area, alpine (downhill) skiing and snowboarding are great forms of exercise and loads of fun. For an even better workout, try the Nordic (cross-country) variety.

* **Dancing.** Particularly fun in a group, dancing—whether country line dancing, swing, salsa, hip-hop, ballroom dancing, ballet, or some other form—is a great way to work out.

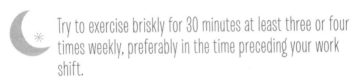

Try to exercise briskly for 30 minutes at least three or four times weekly, preferably in the time preceding your work shift.

Yoga is another form of exercise that may benefit night-shift nurses. Yoga helps reduce stress; maintain muscle strength and flexibility; and decrease weight, systolic and diastolic blood pressure, cholesterol, and triglyceride levels (Li & Goldsmith, 2012; Pal, et al., 2011; Roland, Jakobi, & Jones, 2011). In addition, taking yoga three times per week has been found to boost GABA levels, translating to improved mood and decreased anxiety (Haupt, 2010). (GABA, short for gamma amino-butyric acid, is a chief inhibitory neurotransmitter in the central nervous system.) Yoga classes are offered at many fitness centers and local gymnasiums. Once yoga techniques and poses are learned, they can be practiced at home if you have a simple yoga mat.

Whatever activity you choose, keep in mind that each exercise session should include warm-up, stretching, conditioning, and cool-down periods. In addition, the ACSM (2009; 2010) uses the mnemonic of FITT (frequency, intensity, time, and type) to establish exercise prescriptions:

* **Frequency.** The ACSM recommends that you perform aerobic exercise at least three to five days per week.

* **Intensity.** Exercise should be moderate (in which you experience a noticeable increase in heart rate and breathing) five days per week or vigorous (in which you experience a substantial increase in heart rate and breathing) three days per week.

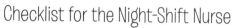

Checklist for the Night-Shift Nurse

The following checklist is designed to help you assess whether your current activity levels are adequate for your needs. Check any of the following boxes that describe your current state.

❏ Feelings of stress (headaches, stomach problems)

❏ Findings from a physical checkup that show an elevated body mass index (BMI)

❏ Findings from a physical checkup that show new onset of diabetes

❏ Feelings of chronic fatigue

❏ Feelings of moodiness

❏ More than two hours of TV watched per day

❏ No physical activity per week

❏ More activity on off days than preceding or following work

❏ Feelings of enjoyment when performing a physical activity

Evaluate the boxes you checked. If you checked any of the first seven, then you might benefit from including exercise in your schedule. Use the ACSM FITT guidelines to help determine your exercise program. Also, establish systems that would increase your activity level. Those systems could include partnering with others, making more time for yourself, learning locations of the closest gyms, or choosing activities that are of the most interest to you.

* **Time.** Moderate workouts should last at least 30 minutes, five days a week, for a total of 150 minutes. Vigorous workouts should last at least 20 to 30 minutes, three days a week, for a total of 75 minutes.

* **Type.** Exercise should be a combination of the aerobic (cardiovascular) and muscular (resistance) variety. Examples of cardiovascular exercise include walking, running, hiking, cycling, aqua aerobics, spinning, dancing, skiing, racquet sports, etc. Examples of resistance exercises include weight train-

ing with dumbbells or machines or exercises with resistance bands. Isometric exercises (muscles being used in opposition) are other examples of resistance exercises.

Getting Started

Hopefully you're already exercising, but if you're reading this chapter there's a good chance you're not. This is a good time to begin! Here are some steps you can take to get your exercise program off the ground:

* **Talk to your health care provider.** As mentioned, it's important that you check with your health care provider before embarking on any new exercise routine. This is especially important if you have any preexisting medical conditions.

* **Scope out your exercise options.** The preceding section covered some options for exercising, from walking to kayaking to yoga and beyond. What exercise options are available to you in your area? Do you live near a ski area? If so, consider snow skiing. Is there a state park nearby? Then hiking or kayaking might be for you.

* **If you find that exercise options are too confusing, begin with walking.** According to the American Heart Association, it's "the simplest, positive change you can make to effectively improve your heart health" (2013).

* **Find a gym.** A great place to start is your local YMCA. In addition to offering classes, pools, and weight and cardio equipment, many YMCAs offer programs in conjunction with health care centers to assist in the prevention of obesity, diabetes, heart disease, and cancer.

* **Take the plunge.** To quote Nike, "Just Do It."

FROM THE TRENCHES

The YMCA is actually attached to our hospital (there is a bridge to get to the YMCA from the main hospital). Employees are encouraged to engage in more healthy lifestyles and this is one way to do that! The YMCA opens at 5 a.m. daily. There are several Summa Health System staff members on the advisory board of the YMCA (myself included), so this has enhanced communication issues. Because Summa employees get a discounted rate, it has been a win-win situation for both the YMCA and Summa employees to take advantage of the facilities.

–Barbara Brunt, MA, MN, RN-BC, NE-BC

 Remember: If you only have time to exercise twice a week, do it. Some exercise is better than no exercise!

* **Develop a routine or system.** It may be easier to devise a specific routine or system — for example, going to the gym every evening before your shift or partnering with friends. Eventually, routine becomes a habit, which decreases the likelihood you'll skip.

FROM THE TRENCHES

I find ways to build exercise into my routine. I don't own a car because I am fortunate enough to live in Chicago with its amazing public transit system (and I have a car-sharing membership and a couple of friends with cars who let me borrow them if I'm in a pinch), so I commute to work via bike and bus (all of Chicago's buses have bike racks), which involves at least two miles of bike riding every work day. On my off days, my lifestyle is an active one—either taking nature walks with my girlfriend, gardening, or otherwise getting around running errands via bike and bus.

–Michael Bennett, MSN, RN, ANP-BC, GNP-BC

FROM THE TRENCHES

For me personally, I would ride my bike into work on nights. I never had to worry about biking in the dark and the ride home actually really helped me to sleep. It also gave me time in the sunlight, which definitely did something for my mood as well.

–Cynthia LaFond, BSN, RN, CCRN

One more thing: You don't have to do all your exercise all at once. Here's what the Mayo Clinic suggests (2011):

Broaden how you think of exercise and find ways to fit activity into your routine. Add small amounts of physical activity throughout your day. For example, take the stairs instead of the elevator. Park a little farther away from your work to fit in a short walk.

If you're just getting started working out, do what you enjoy and start off slowly. If you haven't worked out in years, start exercising 10-15 minutes, a few days a week. Try different exercises to see what you enjoy. As you become fitter, you can increase the duration, intensity, and frequency of your workouts.

FROM THE TRENCHES

I struggled with exercise for quite a while, but find that a quick walk, gym session, or stretching can help me wake up before work. [When I'm off], I can do longer workouts in the middle of the night after everyone has gone to bed.

–June Rolph, BSN, RN

Exercising at Work

Just because you're at work doesn't mean you can't get a bit of exercise. For example, if you're lucky enough to be able to leave your nursing unit during a shift, taking a "lunchtime" stroll can be mentally and physically invigorating. You can also do lunges up and down the halls. In addition, taking the stairs to other units or various levels of the parking garage will burn extra calories. Moving about may also help you combat fatigue: "Keep yourself moving throughout your shift to help your mind stay awake and active. Sitting idle will decrease your blood flow and cause you to become sluggish" (Wong, 2012).

 Using a pedometer or step counter can help make you acutely aware of the distance you travel each day. Taking 8,000–10,000 steps per day equates to being "somewhat active." Taking more than 12,500 steps per day equates to being "highly active" (Roitman & LaFontaine, 2012).

FROM THE TRENCHES

It's the middle of the night on my unit. I come out of my patient's room to find the nurses' stations empty. My first concern is that a clinical emergency may be occurring. After seeing both of the code carts undisturbed, I know just where to find everyone. I tiptoe down the center hallway and, sure enough, I see my fellow coworkers actively participating in lunges and squats. Yes, I am lucky enough to work on a unit that values exercise and promotes healthy practices both in and out of work. Our night shift has become particularly concerned with exercise patterns, and we have held such contests as the 60-day Insanity workouts and Biggest Loser competitions, and have even organized events outside of work, including a hula-hooping class, rock-climbing at a local climbing wall, yoga classes, and running groups. Instead of falling into the all-too-common night-shift patterns of overeating and decreased *exercise, we have nutritious meal nights and cheer each other on in our attempts to become healthier and happier nurses. As I get in line to start the jumping jacks I realize something: No matter how tired I am, there's nowhere I'd rather be.*

–Jolene Schaeffer, RN

Here are a few other simple exercises you can perform to alleviate stress and improve fitness:

* **Work the glutes.** While charting, do toe rises and squeeze your glutes together. Hold for a few seconds and then relax. Repeat as tolerated (Durning, 2011). If you are near a desk, hold on to the desk and slowly lift one leg and hold it in place for about 15 seconds. Switch legs and repeat.

* **Work the arms.** While holding full water bottles, extend the arms up to shoulder height, hold for a few seconds, and then lower them. Repeat 10 to 15 times (Durning, 2011). Another idea is to utilize therapy bands. Holding the band with both hands, raise it above the head. Then, with the right hand, pull the band down to the right shoulder height while keeping the left hand up in the air. Switch sides. Repeat as tolerated.

* **Work the legs.** Slowly lift one leg out straight to hip level, hold it in place for approximately 15 seconds, and relax. Alternate legs and repeat the sequence as tolerated (Durning, 2011).

* **Do squats.** Sneak in a few squats while you are in a patient's room. While you are emptying the urinary drainage bag, squat while keeping your back straight. Hold that position for a few seconds and then slowly return to a standing position.

Some organizations provide an on-site fitness center for employees, often for free. This can really help employees get the exercise they need!

Partner with a coworker or buddy to keep you on track with your exercise.

FROM THE TRENCHES

The Nursing Night Council, a nursing shared leadership council at University of Texas Medical Branch (UTMB) in Galveston, Texas, partnered with the Employee Health and Wellness Team. The Night Council's strategic plan is to promote a healthy work environment. As part of an overall wellness plan, the Nursing Night Council was concerned about the lack of organized physical activity during their work hours of 7 p.m. to 7 a.m. Increasing physical activity in the workplace can make existing wellness programs more comprehensive and is a great way to start a new program. At work, employees are often presented with a choice between taking the stairs and taking an elevator. Choosing the stairs instead of the elevator is a quick way for people to add physical activity to their day.

The UTMB Health Promotion team along with the Nursing Night Council committed to having one event per month during the hours of 6 p.m. to 8 p.m. The first "Caught in the Stairs" event in September 2012 rewarded 120 employees with a bottle of ice water and a tee shirt for walking the stairs. The second event in October 2012 "caught" 150 employees in the stairs. In November, a full day of physical activity events was planned "and started at 6:30 a.m. and ended at 8 p.m. The members found these activities enhanced teamwork, morale, and productivity.

–Barbara Bonificio, MS, RN-BC; Elvia Gomez, BSN, RN-BC; Souby George, MSN, RN; and Amy Carroll, MSN, RN, CCRN

References

American College of Sports Medicine (ACSM). (2009). *ACSM's resource manual for guidelines for exercise testing and prescription* (6th ed.). Philadelphia, PA: Wolters Kluwer | Lippincott Williams & Wilkins.

American College of Sports Medicine (ACSM). (2010). *ACSM's guidelines for exercise testing and prescription* (8th ed.). Philadelphia, PA: Wolters Kluwer | Lippincott Williams & Wilkins.

American Heart Association. (2013, February 26). American Heart Association guidelines for physical activity. Retrieved from http://www.heart.org/HEARTORG/GettingHealthy/PhysicalActivity/StartWalking/American-Heart-Association-Guidelines-for-Physical-Activity_UCM_307976_Article.jsp

Bumgardner, W. (2008). Walking reduces breast cancer risk. *About.com.* Retrieved from http://walking.about.com/cs/cancerprevention/a/bcnursestudy.htm

da Nobrega, L. (2005). The subacute effects of exercise: Concept, characteristics, and clinical implications. *Exercise Sports Science Review, 33*(2), 84-87.

Durning, M. (2011). Top 10 at-work stress relief exercises for nurses. *Scrubs.* Retrieved from http://scrubsmag.com/top-ten-stress-relief-exercises-for-nurses/

Eberly, R., & Feldman, H. (2010). Obesity and shift work in the general population. *The Internet Journal of Allied Health Sciences and Practice, 8*(3). Retrieved from http://ijahsp.nova.edu/articles/Vol8Num3/pdf/feldman.pdf

Haupt, A. (2010, September 24). Benefits of yoga: How different types affect health. *US News Health.* Retrieved from http://health.usnews.com/health-news/diet-fitness/fitness/articles/2010/09/24/benefits-of-yoga-how-different-types-affect-health

Hu, F. B., Stamfer, M. J., Colditz, G. A., Ascherio, A., Rexrode, K. M., Willett, W. C., & Manson, J. E. (2000). Physical activity and risk of stroke in women. *Journal of the American Medical Association, 283*(22), 2961-2967.

Knowler, W. C., Barrett-Conner, E., Fowler, S. E., Hamman, R. F., Lachin, J. M., Walker, E. A., & Nathan, D. M. (2002). Reduction in the incidence of type 2 diabetes with lifestyle intervention or metformin. Diabetes Prevention Program Research Group. *New England Journal of Medicine, 346*(6), 393-403.

Li, A. W., & Goldsmith, C. A. (2012). The effects of yoga on anxiety and stress. *Alternative Medicine Review, 17*(1), 21-35.

Mahoney, S. (2011). Exercise and cortisol levels. *Livestrong.com.* Retrieved from http://www.livestrong.com/article/86687-exercise-cortisol-levels/

Manson, J. E., Hu, F. B., Rich-Edwards, J. W., Colditz, G. A., Stamfer, M. J., Willett, W. C....Hennekens, C. H. (1999). A prospective study of walking as compared with vigorous exercise in the prevention of coronary heart disease in women. *New England Journal of Medicine, 341*(9), 650-658. Retrieved from http://www.nejm.org.proxy.uchicago.edu/doi/pdf/10.056/NEJM1990826340904

Mayo Clinic. (2011). Depression and exercise: Exercise eases symptoms. Retrieved from http://www.mayoclinic.com/health/depression-and-exercise/MH00043

Nieman, D. (2005). Can exercise help me sleep better? *ACSM's Health & Fitness Journal, 9*(3), 6-7.

Pal, A., Srivastava, N., Tiwari, S., Verma, N. S., Narain, V. S., Agrawal, G. G....Kumar, K. (2011). Effect of yogic practices on lipid profile and body fat composition in patients of coronary artery disease. *Complementary Therapies in Medicine, 19*(3), 122-7.

Porter, L. (2010, July 19). How does exercise improve bone density? *Livestrong.com*. Retrieved from www.livestrong.com/article/178849-how-does-exercise-improve-bone-density/

Roitman, J., & LaFontaine, T. (2012). *The exercise professional's guide to optimizing health: Strategies for preventing and reducing chronic disease.* Philadelphia, PA: Lippincott Williams & Wilkins.

Roland, K. P., Jakobi, J. M., & Jones, G. R. (2011). Does yoga engender fitness in older adults? A critical review. *Journal of Aging & Physical Activity, 19*(1), 62-79. Retrieved from http://journals.humankinetics.com/japa-pdf-articles?DocumentScreen=Detail&ccs=6408&cl=21047

U. S. Department of Health and Human Services, Centers for Disease Control and Prevention. (2011). Physical activity and health: The benefits of physical activity. Retrieved from www.cdc.gov/physicalactivity/everyone/health/index.html

Wong, M. (2012). 9 survival tips for night nurses. *healthecareers Network*. Retrieved from http://www.healthecareers.com/article/9-survival-tips-for-night-shift-nurses/169114

Yusuf, S., Hawken, S., Ounpuu, S., Dans, T., Avezum, A., Lanas, F....Lisheng, L. (2004). Effect of potentially modifiable risk factors associated with myocardial infarction in 52 countries (The INTERHEART Study): Case-control study. *Lancet, 364*(9438), 937-952.

Happiness is not a matter of intensity
but of balance, order, rhythm and harmony.

-Thomas Merton

Work/Life Balance

IN THIS CHAPTER

Fostering a healthy work environment

A healthy personal life

Finding balance with the wheel of life

These days, both day and night nurses seek greater work/life balance. In its broadest sense, work/life balance "is defined as a satisfactory level of involvement or 'fit' between the multiple roles in a person's life" (Hudson, 2005).

Why is work/life balance important to nurses? As Terry Chase, MA, ND, RN explains, "Nurses who are out of balance may find that their attention to detail starts to slack, that they are being short with patients and coworkers, that they have a lack of energy, their sleep patterns are interrupted, they lose or gain weight, they look fatigued and they feel like they are leading a passionless existence" (Krischke, 2012). In contrast, notes another nurse leader, Colleen Halberg, MSN, RN, FACHE, "When I am in balance, I am focused, I can accomplish a lot and I can work 10- to 12-hour days with ease, I am able to stay in a positive frame of mind, I sleep well and I feel that I am managing my schedule, rather than my schedule managing me" (Krischke, 2012).

People's perceptions of work/life balance are very subjective. For some, a good balance might simply mean a shorter workweek; for others, balance might be achievable if their job involves less stress. In other words, balance is achieved in different ways for different people. Note, too, that for any one person, work/life balance is achieved through the "right" combination of participation in paid work and other aspects of their lives, a combination that may change in different phases of a person's life.

Today's health care organizations are seeking simultaneously to increase employee satisfaction, increase employee retention, and improve patient outcomes. Fortunately, these goals are not at cross-purposes. Indeed, they are quite well aligned: "Maximizing one's satisfaction as an employee benefits both individual and employer" (Cipriano, 2007). According to Krischke, "Nurses must be attentive to caring for themselves; this will allow them to find a balance between their work life and personal life, which rejuvenates them and allows them to be the best nurses they can be" (2012).

This chapter shows how organizations can improve nurse satisfaction and retention through healthy work environments, and how nurses can improve their satisfaction through work/life balance, even when working the night shift.

Fostering a Healthy Work Environment

Fostering a healthy work environment is essential for nurses—both day and night shifts—to achieve work/life balance. A healthy work environment is also critical for successful nurse recruitment and retention and for the quality of patient care.

But just what is a healthy work environment? Healthy work environments "are characterized by a high level of trust between management and employees; by employees who treat each other in a respectful manner; by an organizational culture that supports skilled communication and collaboration; and by a climate in which employees feel emotionally and physically safe" (Kupperschmidt, Kientz, Ward & Reinholz, 2010). Groff Paris and Terhaar put it this way: "A healthy practice environment is characterized by an engaged nursing staff who exercise control over nursing-related issues, ground their practice in the evidence, and collaborate with colleagues from diverse disciplines" (2010).

Maslow's Hierarchy of Inborn Needs

Groff Paris and Terhaar (2010) align the notion of a healthy work environment with Maslow's Hierarchy of Inborn Needs, which conceptualized human needs as a pyramid with five levels in ascending order. (At the base of Maslow's pyramid are psychologic needs, with safety needs, needs for belonging, needs for esteem, and needs for self-actualization comprising the subsequent layers.) For Groff Paris and Terhaar, nurses' basic needs, such as schedule breaks, workflow, and on-call and overtime expectations, form the base of the pyramid. On the second tier are nurse-to-patient ratios, physician/nurse relationships, acuity, technology, and daily hassles. The next tier is composed of job embeddedness, teamwork, collaboration, communication, and cohesion, while autonomy, empowerment, decision-making ability, and control over practice comprise the pyramid's apex. Groff Paris and Terhaar note, "Applying this model to nursing practice suggests that when nurses do not feel that their basic practice environment needs are being met, they will be less motivated and less likely to progress to the higher-level functions" (2010). They continue: "Maslow's theory suggests that once nurses' basic needs are met, their focus will shift toward achieving higher-level needs, including their sense of belonging, self-esteem, and self-actualization" (2010).

The AACN Standards for a Healthy Work Environment

In 2001, the American Association of Critical-Care Nurses (AACN) committed itself to fostering healthy work environments that support and promote excellence in patient care wherever acute and critical care nurses practice. According to the AACN:

> There is mounting evidence that unhealthy work environments contribute to medical errors, ineffective delivery of care, and conflict and stress among health professionals. Negative, demoralizing and unsafe conditions in workplaces cannot be allowed to continue. The creation of healthy work environments is imperative to ensure patient safety, enhance staff recruitment and retention, and maintain an organization's financial viability (AACN, 2005).

The AACN identified six evidence-based standards for ensuring a healthy work environment and, as a result, move the organization toward the goals of professional satisfaction and patient outcomes. All six standards are essential, with each contributing to the overall development and sustainment of a healthy work environment. Excluding any of the six would reduce an organization's ability to attain a healthy work environment.

The AACN standards for establishing and sustaining healthy work environments are as follows (2005):

* **Skilled communication:** Nurses' communication skills should be as strong as their clinical skills.

* **True collaboration:** Nurses must be relentless in their pursuit of true collaboration.

* **Effective decision-making:** Nurses must act as full partners in developing policy, directing and evaluating clinical care, and leading organizations.

* **Appropriate staffing:** Staffing must effectively match patient needs and nurse competencies.

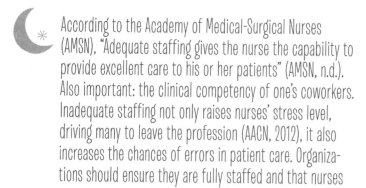

According to the Academy of Medical-Surgical Nurses (AMSN), "Adequate staffing gives the nurse the capability to provide excellent care to his or her patients" (AMSN, n.d.). Also important: the clinical competency of one's coworkers. Inadequate staffing not only raises nurses' stress level, driving many to leave the profession (AACN, 2012), it also increases the chances of errors in patient care. Organizations should ensure they are fully staffed and that nurses are not pressured to take extra shifts or work overtime.

* **Meaningful recognition:** Nurses must be recognized and recognize others for the value they bring to the organization.

* **Authentic leadership:** Nurse leaders must commit to the goal of a healthy work environment, practice it, and engage others in its achievement.

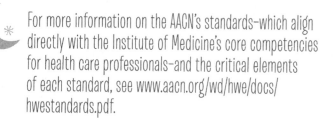

For more information on the AACN's standards–which align directly with the Institute of Medicine's core competencies for health care professionals–and the critical elements of each standard, see www.aacn.org/wd/hwe/docs/hwestandards.pdf.

Becoming a Skilled Communicator

The importance of being a skilled communicator cannot be overemphasized. Indeed, "Professional nurses have an ethical mandate to become skilled communicators to enhance their ability to interact respectfully with all team members and to attain and maintain healthy work environments" (Kupperschmidt, et al., 2010). Failure to communicate properly can also lead to errors in patient care.

One way to become more skilled at communicating is to practice the Five-Factor Model for Becoming a Skilled Communicator. According to this model, skilled communicators must do the following (Kupperschmidt, et al., 2010):

* **Become aware of self deception.** This involves acknowledging misperceptions that are favorable or that enable you to ignore that a problem exists.

* **Become reflective.** This is the process of pondering the meaning of an experience; deriving meaning from past or current experiences in order to guide future behavior; and questioning oneself to better understand situations.

* **Become authentic.** This is a process of self-discovery. It involves understanding your purpose, being self-disciplined, living according to your professional values, practicing with heart, and developing enduring relationships. "Becoming authentic includes a willingness to solicit, receive, and act upon feedback" (Kupperschmidt et al., 2010).

* **Become mindful.** This means developing a heightened awareness of both verbal and nonverbal communication, staying present, and acknowledging and accepting your own thoughts and feelings as they are. Being mindful can also mean "that between the stimulus and response, a nurse can choose to respond positively or react negatively. The nurse who is becoming mindful remains with the current experience without a spill-over of bad feelings from prior interactions" (Kupperschmidt et al., 2010).

> * **Become candid.** Speak purposefully, frankly, and without bias. Speak- and hear-the truth. Unfortunately, due to such fears as job retribution and social retribution, nurses in today's turbulent work environments may be hesitant to speak candidly. "Becoming candid can only happen in environments where nurses feel there is sufficient trust" (Kupperschmidt et al., 2010).
>
> By practicing these behaviors, nurses can engage in private introspection and become skilled communicators.

Of course, it's not enough for the AACN to develop these standards. It's equally critical that organizations adopt them. To that end, the AACN has issued a call to action for health professionals, health care organizations, and the AACN and broader nursing community (2005):

* Nurses and all health professionals are challenged to embrace the personal obligation to participate in creating healthy work environments; develop relationships in which individuals hold themselves and others accountable to professional behavioral standards; and follow through until effective solutions have been realized.

* Health care organizations are challenged to adopt and implement these standards as essential and nonnegotiable for all; establish the organizational systems and structures required for successful education, implementation, and evaluation of the standards; and demonstrate behaviors by example at every level of the organization.

* The AACN and the broader nursing community are challenged to bring to national attention the urgency and importance of healthy work environments; promote these standards as essential to establishing and sustaining healthy work environments; and develop resources to support individuals, organizations, and health systems in successfully adopting the standards and recognizing and publicizing their successes.

Additional Ideas for Fostering a Healthy Work Environment

Who is responsible for fostering a healthy work environment?
Everyone is! That said, the organization must ensure that resources
are allocated to support initiatives and the structures needed to create
the healthy work environment. That means putting into place policies
designed to help employees achieve a balance between their work and
personal commitments. Here are some specific policies that can aid in
this:

* **Offer flexible scheduling.** "Flexibility in scheduling is often
  cited as one of the biggest contributors to a better work/life
  balance" (Larson, 2012). Indeed, this desire is so pervasive, it
  was addressed in a March, 2010 report from the President's
  Council of Economic Advisers, which noted that "American
  workers increasingly need to balance employment with other
  responsibilities" (Executive Office of the President Council
  of Economic Advisers, 2010). Employers who offer flexibility
  in their scheduling and in the number of hours employees
  work not only help their employees achieve work/life balance,
  "They often realize reduced rates of absenteeism and turnover, as well as improvement in productivity and their ability
  to attract and retain workers" (Larson, 2012). As an added
  benefit, employers should have plans in place to accommodate staff members experiencing a family emergency or other
  unplanned personal issue.

* **Offer adequate pay.** As noted by the American Nurses Association (ANA), employers must provide nurses with "sufficient compensation and appropriate staffing systems that foster a safe and healthful environment in which the registered
  nurse does not feel compelled to seek supplemental income
  through overtime, extra shifts, and other practices" (2006).
  This not only helps to alleviate problems associated with
  worker fatigue, but undoubtedly contributes to the work/life
  balance of employees.

FROM THE TRENCHES

The transition to working night shift for a [new-to-practice] RN can be anxiety-producing and overwhelming. The nurse residents often ask questions about how-to strategies on getting the right amount of sleep, what to eat on night shift, and maintaining a healthy work-life balance while working when the rest of their world is sleeping. Using stories and providing practical approaches, the nurse residency program curriculum provides an additional layer of support for achieving a balance while providing safe care. In one of the seminars, the new-to-practice RN completes a self-care assessment and also gains insight into resources on the following:

- *ANA Healthy Nurse Campaign*

- *Exercise*

- *Nutrition*

- *Meditation*

- *Symptoms of fatigue and burnout*

- *Managing stress*

What we have found is most powerful for this component of the program is the comfort the nurse receives in knowing that the organization clearly recognizes and supports each and every individual nurse's well-being as an integral part of providing excellent patient care.

–Beth A. Smith, MSN, RN, UCH/AACN
Nurse Residency Program Coordinator

FROM THE TRENCHES

The Nurse Residency Program helped prepare me for night shift through sharing stories and having an understanding of what to expect…It's reassuring to know that people are there to help and support you through the adjustment.

–Meghan Delaney, BSN, RN, new-to-practice RN

* **Empower nurses.** Nurses must be given clinical autonomy— "the freedom to act on what you know; to make responsible decisions in the nursing sphere, and interdependent decisions in that sphere of practice where nursing overlaps with other disciplines" (Kramer & Schmalenberg, 2008). In addition, nurses should be given "control over their practice when they are able to be a part of decision making in policies and personnel issues" (AMSN, n.d.). As noted by Groff Paris and Terhaar, "Perceptions of empowerment increase when nurses perceive they have control over practice" (2010).

* **Foster collegiality.** Good relationships among nurses, as well as between nurses and other members of the health care team, are "the key to improved patient care. It also decreases nurses' stress levels and increases retention" (AMSN, n.d.).

* **Celebrate.** Work shouldn't be all drudgery. To help foster teamwork and the interpersonal relationships that are critical to the success of any unit, health care organizations should host regular celebrations. These might be to mark certain holidays or birthdays, or to honor a particular staff member's achievements. Celebrations could even be combined with educational opportunities.

It's important that members of the night shift have the same opportunities to celebrate as their day-shift counterparts. For example, at the Hospital of the University of Pennsylvania, where Therese Rutyna, BSN, RN, works, "Any party or celebration on day shift also occurs on night shift on the same day so all staff have the opportunity to celebrate." In addition Rutyna notes, "During Nurses Week events and celebrations, day and night shifts mirror each other."

FROM THE TRENCHES

Night-shift grand rounds at the Hospital of the University of Pennsylvania are both educational and social events. The monthly meetings are scheduled strictly for the night shift and repeated twice to offer a chance for everyone to participate. The topics cover everything from "Leading Through Change" to "What Is Body Language." Staff come to a central location, enjoy some food and conversation before the educational program, then meet with Victoria Rich, our CNE, or her designee to "chat." Staff are always comfortable speaking with Dr. Rich as she has been very accessible to them from the beginning. The style is open forum for this part of the evening. Feedback is extremely positive as night shift is never forgotten in terms of education or having a voice in the organization.

–Patricia Toth, MSN, RN

* **Support nurses' education.** Because education correlates strongly with quality patient care and job satisfaction (and by extension, recruitment and retention), it's imperative that organizations support their employees' efforts to obtain additional education, including continuing education, internships, educational courses, and degrees. This support may be in the form of making education available (for both day- and night-shift workers), offering financial assistance, and rewarding those who obtain education. For example, as Therese Rutyna,

BSN, RN reports, "Our hospital does a great job in providing educational opportunities to the night shift. They hold monthly grand rounds for both RNs and CNAs. Each month has a teaching topic and opportunity to earn continuing education hours." In addition, "For those in school the schedule committee makes sure an employee has either the night before, the night of, or both off to ensure attendance at class."

FROM THE TRENCHES

At the University of Minnesota Amplatz Children's Hospital in Minneapolis, our night nurses have a party every Sunday. The party is unit based and occurs during the shift. They identify different themes and everyone participates and brings a dish to share. We (and they) believe it makes them a stronger team.

We also have an annual celebration of clinical outcomes. The celebration occurs on every shift so the night nurses have the opportunity to participate and have their contributions acknowledged during their shift.

–Meri Beth Kennedy, MS, RN

* **Provide exercise facilities.** To help employees stay fit and maintain work/life balance, consider providing free exercise facilities on site. For example, as noted by Kathy Alkire, BSN, RN, "Our hospital foundation board donated an exercise room for employees complete with treadmill, bike, weight machine, free weights and other equipment to ensure employees stay fit."

FROM THE TRENCHES

One of the ways we've tried to help with staff resiliency is by providing anticipatory guidance. One year, we focused on staff resiliency for our departmental annual competency (session) and incorporated experiential components including mindfulness-based stress reduction, yoga, and music. For our nurse residents, we have provided training in stress management and self-care with the intent of decreasing compassion fatigue.

–Susan Heitzman, MS, RN, CACNS-BC; Bridget Doak, PhD, MT-BC; and Jennifer Encinger, MSW, LICSW

* **Encourage breaks.** Night-shift charge nurses should pay close attention to their colleagues and schedule breaks as needed to help prevent them from "hitting the wall" physically, emotionally, or both (Trimble, n.d.). Although some nurses may be reluctant to briefly set aside their responsibilities in order to recharge, doing so will enable them to maintain higher levels of concentration and performance (Groff Paris & Terhaar, 2010).

FROM THE TRENCHES

One big initiative at the Hospital of the University of Pennsylvania was the foundation of a Center for Nursing Renewal that focuses on promotion of clinical wellness, as well as a space for mental and physical relaxation. This initiative was a vision of our Chief Nurse Executive, Victoria L. Rich, PhD, RN, FAAN, to support nurses in providing excellence in patient care through self-care. The Center for Nursing Renewal houses a relaxation room with massage chairs, a meditation room, a lending library, computer café, and conference room space. In addition to the space, it has opened the doors for many staff to facilitate and participate in classes such as yoga, Zumba, and Reiki.

–Beth A. Smith, MSN, RN

* **Minimize hassles.** As noted by Groff Paris and Terhaar, "Daily 'hassles,' such as 'hunting and gathering activities'"—for example, taking the time to find medication and supplies—"deter nurses from meaningful patient care" (2010). Groff Paris and Terhaar continue: "These basic stressors can threaten patient safety and adversely affect the nurses' perceptions of their practice environment" (2010).

* **Offer concierge services.** Offering employees easy access to services such as dry cleaning, gift wrapping, and so on is a great way to help them maintain work/life balance.

* **Offer an employee assistance program.** Often, events in a nurse's personal life upset the work/life balance. When that happens, employers can help by providing employee assistance programs. An employee assistance program offers services ranging from counseling to legal advice to the location of local resources for child and elder care (Krischke, 2012).

* **Accommodate night nurses' schedules.** Asking night-shift workers to attend meetings during the day shift is like asking day-shift workers to come in at midnight. To ensure that night-shift staff have the opportunity to recharge away from work, organizations must accommodate their schedules by hosting meetings during their shift. This might mean holding the same meeting multiple times, to ensure everyone has an opportunity to attend. For example, as Therese Rutyna, BSN, RN describes, "The nurse manager and/or the assistant nurse manager come in at 5 a.m. to hold monthly staff meetings with the night-shift staff. This is done three days in a row so most of the night-shift staff has a chance to attend."

FROM THE TRENCHES

Two years ago, we started scheduling meetings specifically for night-shift nurses to get together and discuss topics that were specific to night shift. The whole idea was the result of night nurses who were members of shared governance councils. These nurses were having difficulty making meetings during the day, but wanted to be active and participate in nursing decision-making in the hospital. The night meeting was called "Night Force." The idea was so popular that all disciplines are now invited to participate.

The Night Force meetings were originally every month and now meet every two to three months. They last one hour and are facilitated by two RNs who help follow up on the ideas and recommendations made during the meetings. Normally, there are guests from administration at each meeting discussing some of the topics that were brought up from the last meeting. Some examples of topics discussed are parking, food options at night, housekeeping, and supplies, just to name a few. The directors of each of these departments have been to meetings to answer questions and follow up on topics important to night shift. Refreshments are usually donated by our food and nutrition partners.

Once a person attends a meeting, he or she is added to an email list to receive updates between meetings. The meeting is at 10:15 p.m. The time was set by the members. Normally, there is at least one representative from each area, depending on what is going on and how busy the units are. The staff on the unit covers for the person who attends. That person usually brings input from the unit staff and then relays information back to the staff after the meeting.

–Michelle J. Burns, MSN, RN

FROM THE TRENCHES

Our Night Advisory Council started in 2007 under the leadership of our vice president of nursing and patient-care services. The council is a place where information is shared not only about what the administration is doing, but also about night-staff needs. The night staff started to give presentations to each other about topics of interest to them; one of the first presentations was about night-staff wellness. Later, we had a session about patient wellness at night. The council is seen as an effective forum for the night staff to be recognized and to be involved.

–Carolyn Castelli, MSN, RN, PMHCNS-BC

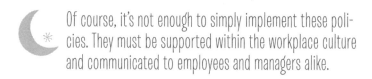

Of course, it's not enough to simply implement these policies. They must be supported within the workplace culture and communicated to employees and managers alike.

A Healthy Personal Life

Even if your employer takes all the steps necessary to create a healthy work environment, you cannot achieve work/life balance if things are lousy in your personal life. In large part, that means you must work hard to stay connected with friends and family members as well as taking time for yourself—no small challenge for those working the night shift! On top of that, you must manage your finances and tend to the minutiae of daily life, running errands, doing chores, and the like. Here are a few tips to help you juggle all these responsibilities and maintain your equilibrium:

* Working the night shift may limit the time you have to spend with friends and family, especially for spontaneous get-togethers. To make sure you stay connected, schedule activities together whenever you can. When you can't get together, make it a point to call friends and extended family to see how they're doing and to share what's going on in your life (Wong, 2012).

* When possible, meet with your kids' teachers. Volunteer as a chaperone for school field trips or as a teacher's aide (Trimble, n.d.).

* Even if you and your spouse and/or other family members are on opposite schedules, try to eat together as often as possible. Your "breakfast" might be their "dinner," and your "dinner" might be their "breakfast."

* Balance work and family life, but build in dedicated time for you.

* Foster a passion for a hobby or something you like to do.

* If you live alone, consider getting a pet. People who have pets are generally happier than those who do not have pets. Pet owners, particularly dog owners, weigh less, are less sedentary, have lower blood pressure and lower cholesterol and triglyceride levels (Arhant-Sudhir, Arhant-Sudhir, & Sudhir, 2011).

FROM THE TRENCHES

Take time for you and your family. Get a massage, facial, manicure, or pedicure, go shopping, find a hobby; do something that makes you feel pampered and relaxed. Enjoy a family outing. Have a date night. Take the kids out for ice cream. Establish family game time. Go out with friends. In order to take care of others, you need to take care of yourself! Sometimes working nights, it is difficult to find the time and energy, but do it!

–Kathy Alkire, BSN, RN

* Take vacations, and not just the kind where you putz around the house for a week. Really get away.

* Find a routine and stick to it. "The body functions better when a routine is followed, and researchers have suggested that following an established routine may decrease depressive symptoms among night workers (Pronitis-Ruotolo, 2001).

FROM THE TRENCHES

For balancing life, family, and relationship needs, the best tip, in my opinion, is clustering shifts together, so as to be able to adjust back to a normal schedule and spend time with them.

–Michael Bennett, MSN, RN, ANP-BC, GNP-BC

* Eat right, exercise, and get enough sleep. As noted by one nurse leader, "People who have to work hard need to be ready to do so and if they aren't refreshing their body and mind they are going to start showing signs of stress" (Krischke, 2012). For more, refer to Chapter 2, "Night Shift, Fatigue, and Sleep," Chapter 4, "Healthful Eating," and Chapter 5, "Exercise Benefits."

* Be financially responsible. If possible, live on the income you would earn by working the day shift rather than relying on your night-shift differential to make ends meet. Instead, "Use your differential income for specific short-term purposes such as debt reduction, extra investment, vacation funds" (Trimble, n.d.).

Finding Balance with the Wheel of Life

 The information in this section appears courtesy of MindTools.com.

If life is busy or all your energy is focused on a special project, you may quickly find yourself "off balance"—not paying enough attention to important areas of your life—which can lead to frustration and intense stress. When that happens, it's time to take a helicopter view of your life so you can bring things back into balance. But how?

To aid in this, use a tool called the wheel of life. Commonly used by professional life coaches, it helps you consider each area of your life, assess what's off balance, and in doing so, identify areas that need more attention. It is called the "wheel of life" because each area of your life is mapped on a circle, like the spoke of a wheel. The wheel of life is powerful because it gives you a vivid visual representation of the way your life is currently, compared with how you'd like it to be. An example of a wheel of life, with a set of sample dimensions, husband/wife, mother/father, manager, colleague, etc., is shown in Figure 6.1. This approach assumes that you will be happy and fulfilled if you can find the right balance of attention for each of these dimensions, and that different areas of your life will need different levels of attention at different times.

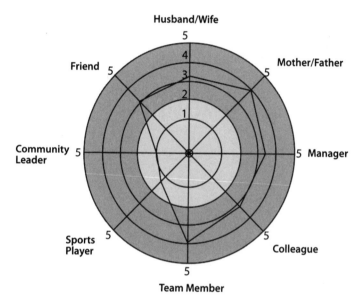

Figure 6.1   The wheel of life.

To create your own wheel of life, follow these steps:

1. Brainstorm the six to eight dimensions of your life that are important for you. These might include the roles you play in life (husband/wife, father/mother, manager, colleague, team member, sports player, community leader, friend, etc.), the areas of life that are important to you (artistic expression, positive attitude, career, education, family, friends, financial freedom, physical challenge, pleasure, public service, etc.),

or a combination of these (or different) things, reflecting the priorities in your life.

2. Write down these dimensions on the blank wheel of life diagram shown in Figure 6.2, one on each spoke.

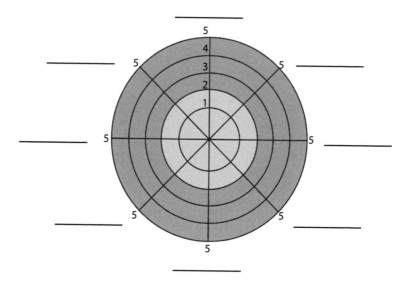

Figure 6.2 Write down the dimensions of your life that are important to you on this blank wheel of life.

3. Assess the amount of attention you're currently devoting to each area. Consider each dimension in turn, and on a scale of 0 (low) to 5 (high), write down the amount of attention you're devoting to that area of your life. Mark each score on the appropriate spoke of your life wheel.

4. Join up the marks around the circle. Does your life wheel look and feel balanced?

5. Consider your ideal level in each area of your life. A balanced life does not mean attaining a 5 in each area; some areas need more attention and focus than others at any one time. Inevitably, you will need to make choices and compromises, as your time and energy are not in unlimited supply!

So the question is, what would the ideal level of attention be for you in each life area?

6. Plot the "ideal" scores around your life wheel. You now have a visual representation of your current life balance and your ideal life balance. What are the gaps? These are the areas of your life that need attention.

Remember, gaps can go both ways. There are almost certainly areas that are not getting as much attention as you'd like. However, there may also be areas where you're putting in more effort than you should. These areas are sapping energy and enthusiasm that may be better directed elsewhere.

7. Once you have identified the areas that need attention, it's time to plan the actions needed to work on regaining balance. Starting with the neglected areas, what do you need to start doing to regain balance? In the areas that currently sap your energy and time, what can you stop doing or reprioritize or delegate to someone else? Make a commitment to these actions by writing them on your wheel of life.

You can use the wheel of life as preparation for goal setting or coaching. It helps identify the areas you want to work on and is a great way of visualizing your current and desired life. Once you are working on improving your life balance, it's also a useful tool for monitoring your life balance as it changes over time.

The wheel of life is a great tool to help you improve your life balance. It helps you quickly and graphically identify the areas in your life to which you want to devote more energy and helps you understand where you might want to cut back. The challenge now is to transform this knowledge and desire for a more balanced life into a positive program of action!

References

Academy of Medical-Surgical Nurses (AMSN). (n.d.). Healthy work environment. Retrieved from http://www.amsn.org/HWE/Characteristics.html

American Association of Colleges of Nursing (AACN). (2012). Nursing shortage. Retrieved from http://www.aacn.nche.edu/media-relations/fact-sheets/nursing-shortage

American Association of Critical-Care Nurses (AACN). (2005). AACN standards for establishing and sustaining healthy work environments. Retrieved from http://www.aacn.org/WD/HWE/Docs/HWEStandards.pdf

American Nurses Association (ANA). (2006). Assuring patient safety: The employers' role in promoting healthy nursing work hours for registered nurses in all roles and settings. *NursingWorld*. Retrieved from http://www.nursingworld.org/MainMenu-Categories/Policy-Advocacy/Positions-and-Resolutions/ANAPositionStatements/Position-Statements-Alphabetically/AssuringPatientSafety.pdf

Arhant-Sudhir, K., Arhant-Sudhir, R., & Sudhir, K. (2011). Pet ownership and cardiovascular risk reduction: Supporting evidence, conflicting data and underlying mechanisms. *Clinical Experimental Pharmacology and Physiology, 38*(11), 734-738. Retrieved from http://onlinelibrary.wiley.com/doi/10.1111/j.1440-1681.2011.05583.x/full

Cipriano, P. (2007). Work/life balance? Yes, please! *American Nurse Today, 2*(8). Retrieved from http://www.americannursetoday.com/article.aspx?id=3754&fid=37

Executive Office of the President Council of Economic Advisers. (2010). Work-life balance and the economics of workplace flexibility. *WhiteHouse.gov*. Retrieved from http://www.whitehouse.gov/files/documents/100331-cea-economics-workplace-flexibility.pdf

Groff Paris, L. & Terhaar, M. (2010). Using Maslow's Pyramid and the National Database of Nursing Quality Indicators to attain a healthier work environment. *OJIN: The Online Journal of Issues in Nursing, 16*(1). Retrieved from http://www.nursingworld.org/MainMenuCategories/ANAMarketplace/ANAPeriodicals/OJIN/TableofContents/Vol-16-2011/No1-Jan-2011/Articles-Previous-Topics/Maslow-and-NDNQI-to-Assess-and-Improve-Work-Environment.aspx

Hudson Global Resources, (Aust) Pty Ltd. (2005). The case for work/life balance: Closing the gap between policy and practice. Retrieved from http://au.hudson.com/Portals/AU/documents/Hudson2020_Work-Life.pdf

Kramer, M., & Schmalenberg, C. (2008). The practice of clinical autonomy in hospitals: 20,000 nurses tell their story. *Critical Care Nurse, 28*(6), 58–71. Retrieved from http://ccn.aacnjournals.org/content/28/6/58.full

Krischke, M. (2012). Nurse leaders offer wisdom on achieving work-life balance. *NurseZone.com*. Retrieved from http://www.nursezone.com/nursing-news-events/more-features/Nurse-Leaders-Offer-Wisdom-on-Achieving-WorkLife-Balance_37400.aspx

Kupperschmidt, B., Kientz, E., Ward, J., & Reinholz, B. (2010). A healthy work environment: It begins with you. *OJIN: The Online Journal of Issues in Nursing, 15*(1). Retrieved from http://www.nursingworld.org/MainMenuCategories/ANAMarketplace/ANAPeriodicals/OJIN/TableofContents/Vol152010/No1Jan2010/A-Healthy-Work-Environment-and-You.html

Larson, J. (2012). More employers helping nurses pursue work-life balance. *NurseZone.com*. Retrieved from http://www.nursezone.com/nursing-news-events/more-news/More-Employers-Helping-Nurses-Pursue-Work%E2%80%93life-Balance_39432.aspx

MindTools. (n.d.). The Wheel of Life. *MindTools*. Retrieved from http://www.mindtools.com/pages/article/newHTE_93.htm

Pronitis-Ruotolo, D. (2001). Surviving the night shift: Making *Zeitgeber* work for you. *American Journal of Nursing, 101*(7). 63–68.

Trimble, T. (n.d.). Night shift survival hints. *Emergency Nursing World*. Retrieved from http://enw.org/NightShift.htm

Wong, M. (2012). 9 survival tips for night nurses. *healthecareers Network*. Retrieved from http://www.healthecareers.com/article/9-survival-tips-for-night-shift-nurses/169114

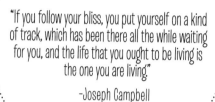

7

"If you follow your bliss, you put yourself on a kind
of track, which has been there all the while waiting
for you, and the life that you ought to be living is
the one you are living."

-Joseph Campbell

Keeping Your Career on Track

IN THIS CHAPTER

Staying visible at work

Learning opportunities

Job options for night-shift nurses

Finding a new job

Night shift is often called the "graveyard shift" or the "dead-end shift," the insinuation being that working nights is a dead-end job, despite the fact that the pay is often higher (indeed, by as much as 20%). This perception occurs because nurses who work the night shift are rarely seen or heard by the "day" people, including administration. Indeed, this "invisibility" is among the chief complaints of those who work the night shift, and it can be terribly frustrating to those nurses who are particularly career minded!

However, this doesn't mean there aren't vibrant roles to assume during the night shift or that doing night work means your career won't advance. Indeed, night-shift nurses are "at an advantage when it comes to raises and promotions. You are not competing with the day workers, of which there are many more than the night shift, so you have more opportunities to climb the promotion ladder" (Rothstein, 2012), especially within roles designated for night shift. Put another way, "If you are highly effective and actually like nights, you may rise to your highest level there and stay forever" (Trimble, n.d.). The fact is, as you'll discover in this chapter, you don't have to move off nights to build a wonderful career.

Staying Visible at Work

As mentioned in Chapter 1, "Advantages, Challenges, and Risks of Night Work," night nurses often feel invisible both to their counterparts on the day shift and to the overall leadership. An unfortunate consequence of this invisibility is career stall, as "invisibility to daytime administrators and power-brokers increases" (Trimble, n.d.).

Getting Involved

As noted by Trimble, "If you seek career-advancement and consistently work nights, you will have to find useful ways to overcome the 'invisibility' of not being frequently seen by administrators and committees. Tasks often tried include coordinating night scheduling, orientation and in-services presented, liaison with EMS, projects, etc." (n.d.).

Ideally, your facility ascribes to the notion of shared governance—that is, the idea that nurses on all shifts, including night shift, participate in decision-making. If so, make it a point to engage. Choose a committee that centers around an area that interests you and get involved (Keefe, 2011). In addition, you must make it a point to routinely attend staff meetings and other unit meetings and make your voice heard, even if it sometimes means coming in early or staying late.

Although you might think that meetings need to be face-to-face, you should also think about using technology to enhance the use of "virtual" committee meetings or project work. You can set a meeting agenda and have discussions in online formats (assuming they are approved by your organization). Discussions can occur over a period of time to allow peers on all shifts to have input on decisions. Likewise, writing publications or creating presentations can also occur through virtual methods. When you realize that you don't need to be sitting in a room at the same time, then you can visualize and implement creative ways of collaborating across shifts.

FROM THE TRENCHES

As a night-shift nurse, one of the greatest challenges I face is staying connected with my colleagues and activities happening in my hospital during the day hours. My advice to anyone who works at night is to try to participate in a select number of activities in order to maintain communication with peers. I say a "select number" because no one can participate in everything that happens in a large facility. You can limit your activities to areas you are truly passionate about. This will help you maintain the spark to make a commitment to be active. I participate on my unit and hospital-wide shared governance councils and attend as many staff meetings as possible. These commitments do require some personal effort. You may have to come in on days off or stay over after a shift, but these sacrifices pay off in the relationships you build with peers. It broadens your network throughout the hospital and, for me, it helps me feel more a part of my institution and the nursing profession.

–Carol V. Cromer, BSN, RNC-OB

Presenting Yourself Professionally

An important part of staying visible is presenting yourself professionally. "Understanding and practicing professionalism will foster self-respect, self-satisfaction, and confidence. It will also help to garner more respect, recognition, and opportunities for you and for all nurses" (Cardillo, 2009).

Professional presentation means, among other things, "dressing in a manner that conveys maturity, seriousness of purpose, and conservative good taste" (Cardillo, 2009). The fact is, how you dress makes a powerful statement about who you are. As noted by Pagana (2008):

> The way you dress supports or detracts from your professional image. It sends a message to others about how you see yourself and how you want to be perceived by others. It sets the stage for what others may expect from you. Most nurses agree that they would like to be viewed as professional, intelligent, and competent. They need to ask themselves if their appearance mirrors that image.

For example, sloppy or inappropriate attire "could imply that you do not respect yourself, that you do not place value on appearance, or that you do not care that your appearance impacts the corporate image" (Pagana, 2008). Moreover, "If nurses dress too casually, patients may question their attention to detail and their professionalism. Patients often associate appearance with trustworthiness or ability" (Pagana, 2008).

For guidance on appropriate attire, "Look how leaders and managers dress in different positions, and model your attire to match theirs...If you are looking to advance your career, dress like the people the next level up" (Pagana, 2008). Here are some general guidelines (Cardillo, 2009; Pagana, 2008):

* Uniforms, lab coats, scrubs, and shoes should be clean, pressed, in good repair, and conservative in appearance.
* Long hair should be pulled back and out of the face.

* Name tags should be visible and readable.
* Tattoos and piercings should not be visible. Not only are these forbidden by many employers, they may be offensive or even frightening to some patients.
* Perfumes or colognes should be applied with great moderation, if at all. Many people are allergic to these scents; as a result, some workplaces do not permit employees to wear them.

Demonstrating Good Communication Skills

Another important way to stay visible is to demonstrate good communication skills, in person-to-person contact, on the phone, and in electronic forms such as email, texts, or pages. "If you've ever received a rude email or been frustrated by an unhelpful reply, you can attest to the fact that these experiences affect your attitude and perception of the person on the other end of the exchange. In the same way, if someone goes above and beyond to answer your question, provide you with useful information, or share resources or contacts, you will have a completely different perception of that person" (Fraser, 2011).

When communicating in writing, remember that the receiver has only your written words to understand your message. It's easy for a message to be misinterpreted when the receiver cannot hear your voice or see your face, both of which provide context to a message. When sending a written message, you might want to read it aloud to yourself as a way of checking what you will be sending.

Here are a few other tips for using these forms of communication:

* Keep your messages simple and to the point. This helps the receiver know what is being conveyed and what action to take.
* When writing messages, refrain from using ALL CAPS or bolded lettering. Both may make the receiver feel as if you are yelling at him or her.

* If you are sending a message that needs a reply within a given time frame, please let the receiver know. If sending an email, use the Subject line to help the receiver prioritize when the message needs to be read and responded to.

* Before sending an email, check that you are sending the message to the correct person(s). Especially when addressing a patient issue, it is important to maintain all Health Insurance Portability and Accountability Act (HIPAA) standards and ensure that patient information is protected.

* If you use abbreviations or acronyms, make sure that they are standard for your organization. Again, this helps ensure that everyone can interpret the message correctly.

* If you write a message while angry, don't send it right away. Save the message as a draft, cool down, and reread the message before sending it. Ask yourself, What is the issue? What is needed? What can I suggest or request? Then determine whether your message provides that information in a clear and direct manner. Although venting can feel good, anger can derail communication. Taking time to calm down and focus on the issue enables you to write a clear communication.

 If you have strong writing skills, consider writing for publication or starting your own blog. This is a great way to garner attention and advance your career.

Communicating face-to-face or via the phone during the night shift can provide its own challenges. Awareness that fatigue compromises communication for all employees at night helps you improve your approach to communication. Remember to maintain professionalism in all communication. Speak politely and clearly and be willing to repeat your statement(s) so the receiver can understand all that you say. In addition, repeat essential information, such as lab values or a critical decision, to ensure that everyone involved has the same understanding of what has been conveyed.

When waking someone during the night—a health care provider, manager, or peer—provide context for your call. For example, you could start with saying who you are and where you are calling from, then begin the request or report. It might take the receiver a few seconds or even minutes to be clear about what the communication is about.

Remember, it is equally important to be clear in text or page messages that might awaken a person. Leaving a simple phone number will not convey the situation to the receiver. Short, clear statements that include your name, phone and/or page number, and clinical unit will help the receiver respond to you in a timely manner.

Change-of-shift reports are a particularly risky time due to fatigue for the offgoing staff. Using a standardized method of reporting helps ensure that key patient information is provided for a safe handoff of patients between the offgoing and oncoming staff. The situation-background-assessment-recommendation (SBAR) technique for communication about a patient's condition can be a helpful reporting tool (Kaiser Permanente of Colorado, 2011). Rounding on your patients with the offgoing staff as part of your reporting process also helps to ensure that relevant information is conveyed.

It's also important to use nonverbal communication—body language—to your best advantage. It's particularly critical to keep your facial expressions in check. For example, "Don't roll your eyes in the presence of patients or staff when a physician or manager says something you don't agree with. Address it in private" (Cardillo, 2009).

As noted in Chapter 6, "Work/Life Balance," the importance of being a skilled communicator cannot be overemphasized. Indeed, "Professional nurses have an ethical mandate to become skilled communicators to enhance their ability to interact respectfully with all team members and to attain and maintain healthy work environments" (Kupperschmidt, Kientz, Ward, & Reinholz, 2010).

For more information about becoming a skilled communicator, refer to Chapter 6. It discusses the Five-Factor Model for Becoming a Skilled Communicator. According to this model, skilled communicators must become aware of self-deception, become reflective, become authentic, become mindful, and become candid. By practicing these behaviors, nurses can engage in private introspection and become skilled communicators (Kupperschmidt et al., 2010).

A Word on Social Media

Recent years have seen a proliferation in the use of social media, including among nurses. Indeed, social media can be a great professional tool. As noted by Robert Fraser, author of *The Nurse's Social Media Advantage*:

> Social media spreads information, enables people to communicate, and facilitates collaboration. When you use Web services, other people can read, listen to, and watch content you produce, as well as read about you in your profiles. These services also make it easier to others to see how you communicate and to directly communicate or collaborate with you.

Social media is also, according to Fraser, "a great platform for nurses to share their expertise with the public and to shed insight into what nurses do and the value they add to the health care system."

Fraser observes that developing a positive reputation online can represent a real opportunity offline. It can help you become known for specific skills or abilities; foster interest among potential employers; secure opportunities to fulfill career goals; and more. "No one, to my knowledge, has ever been fired for developing an online presence as an expert in their field or as an intelligent and hard-working individual" (2011).

That means, of course, that you must avoid cultivating a negative online reputation, as your career and professional reputation may be on the line. If you choose to engage in social media, you'll want to keep some points in mind (Fraser, 2011):

* Find out whether your employer maintains a policy on or related to social media. If it does, "you are required to abide by it when at work or representing your organization" (Fraser, 2011).

* Be aware of the Health Insurance Portability and Accountability Act (HIPAA), which protects patient confidentiality. To avoid breaking this law, never use patient names or identifiers (phone numbers, hospital IDs, etc.); speak about patients in generalities; do not disclose dates or time frames; avoid discussing treatment location; and do not post pictures of patients. Talk about general lessons learned, not specific patient experiences.

* Don't share content that might damage your reputation, "such as pictures of alcohol use, shop talk, criticisms of employers, or questionable posts from friends" (Fraser, 2011).

FROM THE TRENCHES

The Nursing Ethics Interest Group recently set up a Yammer site, which will allow nurses on all shifts to respond to questions related to issues or to join in chat discussions.... Mayo (Clinic) uses Yammer as an internal professional connectivity tool. It is secure and apparently inaccessible to those external (to the organization). There are all kinds of different groups, from "Eating Well at Work" to "Innovation" to "Qualitative Research" to workgroup-specific groups. What I see it most effective for is when someone has a question or problem, they can post a question and have almost immediate answers from people they might not even know exist in the organization.

–Joan Henriksen Hellyer, PhD, RN, and
Anne Miers, MSN, RN, CNRN, ACNS-BC

Learning Opportunities

As you no doubt know, it's not enough to simply earn your nursing degree and obtain your license. As a nurse, you will find yourself in a continuous learning cycle. This might involve furthering your formal education—for example, obtaining a bachelor's degree in nursing, completing an advanced nursing degree program to obtain a master's degree or an advanced practice registered nurse and doctoral degree, or attending in-services and continuing education (CE) contact hour presentations.

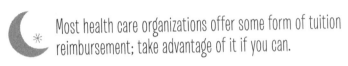

Most health care organizations offer some form of tuition reimbursement; take advantage of it if you can.

The continuous learning cycle may also include regular attendance at nursing seminars and continuing education programs, pursuing clinical certification when appropriate, and reading industry journals (Cardillo, 2009). To keep your career on track, take advantage of available learning opportunities, such as clinical or leadership classes, whenever possible. Be sure to communicate your learning goals—and your accomplishments—to your manager (Claffey, 2011).

FROM THE TRENCHES

Night-shift grand rounds occur twice monthly at 1 a.m. and 3 a.m., during which an in-service is provided for all units to attend. These in-services are provided by the professional development specialists or the clinical nurse specialists. The challenge is coverage at night for nurses to attend a lecture outside their unit. An innovative idea of providing a "road show" allows for increased attendance of clinical nurses and certified nursing assistants for applicable topics. The educational information is condensed to a half hour with a 0.5 CE and snacks to accompany. The charge nurse of each unit is notified a half hour ahead of time to assess time appropriateness and availability of the nurses for the road show. If unavailable, the road show can come back at a more convenient time. When the road show comes to a unit, clinical nurses partake in a central location on the nursing unit. In addition, sister units are notified and join each other in one area to share in the education. These road shows now occur between 11 p.m. and 4 a.m. and allow flexibility for ongoing education with triple the attendance.

–Rebecca Stamm, MSN, RN, CCNS, WCC, CCRN

A Word on Online Courses

While online courses are great for people working the night shift due to the availability of the class that works with your schedule, there are a few downsides. For example, with an online course, "There is no one who will 'prod you along' when you do not complete the assignments on time or post in the discussion sections on a regular basis" (Fant, n.d.). This is in contrast to a traditional class, where students and educators meet regularly, which can help to keep students on track. In addition, technical problems and difficulties navigating the site may arise, which can be a great source of frustration. And because you are not sitting in a classroom with your fellow students, connecting with them in order to network or to obtain help with assignments can be difficult. Even so, online classes can be a great way for night-shift nurses to stay on top of their field.

To determine if online classes fit your student style, talk with the school's recruitment advisor or course advisor to learn how they establish a sense of community within their courses. Many online courses now have time-driven assignments, meaning that you will need to post assignments and comments at regular intervals, as one way of keeping students involved and in active discussion with each other and the instructor.

When deciding on an online program to pursue a formal degree, you might want to connect with students and graduates from that program to learn more about the student experience and then make your best decision. Often, students who were worried about being online students instead of being students in a traditional classroom find that after the initial transition, they adapt well to this method of learning.

Of course, working nights may make it difficult to pursue additional education, as many of the opportunities are likely to occur during the hours you sleep. Even so, it's imperative that you take advantages of learning opportunities whenever possible. That may mean taking courses online, which enable students to complete assignments at almost any time.

Obtaining a BSN

In 1980, the vast majority of registered nurses (RNs) held as their highest educational credential a hospital diploma or an associate degree in nursing. Only 22% of registered nurses held a bachelor's degree. By 2008, however, the number of registered nurses with bachelor's degrees had climbed to 36.8%, with a mere 13.9% of RNs holding a diploma (AACN, 2010).

These days, "More nurse executives are indicating their desire for the majority of their hospital staff nurses to be prepared at the baccalaureate level to meet the more complex demands of today's patient care" (AACN, 2010). As a result, an increasing number of RNs have begun seeking this degree.

Why the new emphasis on the BSN? The AACN (2010) explains:

> The BSN curriculum includes a broad spectrum of scientific, critical-thinking, humanistic, communication, and leadership skills, including specific courses on community health nursing not typically included in diploma or associate-degree tracks. These abilities are essential for today's professional nurse who must be a skilled provider, designer, manager, and coordinator of care. Nurses must make quick, sometimes life-and-death decisions; understand a patient's treatment, symptoms, and danger signs; supervise other nursing personnel; coordinate care with other health providers; master advanced technology; guide patients through the maze of health resources in a community; and teach patients how to comply with treatment and adopt a healthy lifestyle.

The bottom line? "The BSN nurse is prepared for a broader role. The BSN nurse is the only basic nursing graduate preferred to practice in all health care settings—critical care, ambulatory care, public health, and mental health—and thus has the greatest employment flexibility of any entry-level RN" (AACN, 2010). If you work as a nurse but have not earned a BSN, consider going back to school to obtain it. You'll undoubtedly find yourself with more options, whether you switch to the day shift or stick with nights.

For nurses who have been away from school for a few (or many) years, the idea of once again beginning formal study can be daunting. Schools of nursing are very familiar with nurses in this situation and are supportive of their return to academic studies. Do not hesitate to share your concerns with the admission counselor or school representative. You may be surprised by the services that are available to help you with your transition to being a student.

Remember, there is comfort in numbers. Recruit some of your fellow nurses to go back to school with you. Having a buddy or two in the same courses can reduce your anxiety about being new to school! And if technology has you concerned, ask a tech-savvy nurse on your unit to be your technology mentor.

Advanced Degrees

If you seek to advance your career and expand your options, obtaining a master's degree in nursing may well be the way to go. According to the American Association of Colleges of Nursing (AACN), a master's degree in nursing (MSN), which requires 18–24 months of uninterrupted study (more if you opt to fit your studies around your work schedule) "is the educational core that allows advanced practice nurses to work as nurse practitioners, certified nurse midwives, certified clinical nurse specialists, and certified nurse anesthetists" (Dracup, n.d.).

Masters degrees in nursing administration and nursing education are also available.

In addition to clinical coursework as well as classes that focus on a specialty area (such as acute care, geriatrics, pediatrics, etc.), graduate-level programs also include "courses in statistics, research management, health economics, health policy, health care ethics, health promotion, nutrition, family planning, mental health, and the prevention of family and social violence" (Dracup, n.d.). Nursing degrees are continually evaluated and refined, and new majors are created to ensure that nurses are prepared for the future. Think of all the different bodies of knowledge that have developed in the span of your career! Even if you are in your first year, the speed of changes in technology, clinical applications, and patient complexities all influence the evolution in nursing education and programs. Identify what you are curious about and then look for the program of study that fits you!

When looking for the right program, keep in mind that depending on the degree that you are pursuing, field and/or clinical experiences might be required. Traditionally, these occur Monday through Friday during normal "day" hours. However, don't presume that evening or night experiences aren't an option. Some organizations are open to having both field and clinical experiences during "non-day" schedules, especially health care organizations that operate on 24/7 schedules.

Keep in mind that the evolution with nursing education also includes doctoral degrees. Nursing doctoral degrees include both the clinical doctorate, generally referred to as the doctor of nursing practice (DNP), and the traditional or research doctorate, the PhD in nursing. It is important to clearly define your professional goals and compare these goals with both degrees to determine the best option for you. Doctoral degrees are provided in traditional, classroom settings, online, and hybrid (a mixture of classroom and online study) formats.

To find an academic program that's right for you, you'll need to do a bit of research. A great jumping-off spot is the Find Your School section of Johnson & Johnson's site, The Campaign for Nursing's Future. You can find it here: http://www.discovernursing.com/schools. This site also provides a great resource for finding information on scholarships and financial aid.

Ongoing Continuing Education

Continuing education is usually related to new knowledge that is above and beyond the requirements for maintaining your employment. Education and ongoing training or validation of skills and knowledge, such as health provider basic life support certification (BLS), that is required by your employer to maintain your present employment or role is often referred to as "conditions of employment." Not meeting conditions of employment requirements could affect your employment.

Continuing education (CE) that is approved for contact hours should exceed what your employer requires. Many states and all national board certifications have designated CE requirements. It is important to know the specific requirements for your state license as well as your specialty certifications. Access your state nursing professional regulation and licensure website for specific details, as these may be different from one state to the next. You will also want to be knowledgeable about your specialty certification requirements and will be able to access that information at the specific specialty website.

Continuing education is available in in-person, self-study (printed), and online formats, and can be accessed through your place of employment; specialty organizations; local, regional, and national conferences; and direct provider organizations. The cost can range from free to hundreds of dollars for conferences. Carefully research what you are required to do to meet the CE requirements and receive proof of earning CE contact hours.

Certification

A great way to showcase your competence—and your ambition—is to earn professional certifications (Claffey, 2011). As noted by the United States Department of Labor Bureau of Labor Statistics, "Nurses may become credentialed through professional associations in specialties such as ambulatory care, gerontology, and pediatrics, among others. Although certification is usually voluntary, it demonstrates adherence to a higher standard, and some employers may require it" (2012).

For help obtaining certification in a variety of specialties, look to the American Nurses Credentialing Center (ANCC), a subsidiary of the American Nurses Association (ANA). Its internationally renowned Certification Program "enables nurses to demonstrate their specialty expertise and validate their knowledge to employers and patients. Through targeted exams that incorporate the latest nursing-practice standards, ANCC certification empowers nurses with pride and professional satisfaction" (ANCC, n.d.). Obtain more information about certification here: http://www.nursecredentialing. org/certification.aspx. You may also find this link helpful as it has a comprehensive listing of certifications: http://www.nursecredentialing.org/Magnet/Magnet-CertificationForms.

When studying for your certification exam, use as many methods as are helpful to you. These might include taking a certification review course, using note cards, taking practice exams, and participating in buddy or group review sessions.

Many certification exams are available only at computer test sites. Read your testing materials carefully. Note the date, time, place, and what you need to bring. Allow yourself extra time to travel to your test site. Make sure you are well rested for the exam. In other words, do not work the night before the test!

Professional Organizations

Professional organizations for nurses abound. Indeed, a recent Internet search yielded more than 200 such organizations. Some of the organizations focus on a specific nursing specialty, such as neonatal nursing or radiologic and imaging nursing. Others are geared toward nurses of a specific gender or ethnic background. Still others are geographically based, catering to nurses in a particular state.

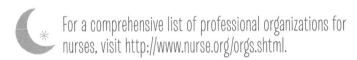

For a comprehensive list of professional organizations for nurses, visit http://www.nurse.org/orgs.shtml.

Becoming active in one or more of these professional organizations can further your knowledge and career. As noted by Cardillo, "Membership provides an opportunity to develop a professional network of peers to share information and best practices, to stay cutting edge with knowledge and information, to create a support system, and to be a vehicle for ongoing personal and professional development" (2009). This can help you find colleagues who share your challenges as a night-shift nurse, and may foster "discussion about best practices to address night-shift problems" (Claffey, 2011).

Job Options for Night-Shift Nurses

Few careers offer as many options for workers as nursing. Indeed, "One of the great strengths of the nursing profession is the variety of career paths, specialties and work environments from which a nurse can choose" (Krischke, 2011). A nurse might choose to work as a clinician, an advance practice nurse, a nurse educator, a nurse administrator, or a nurse researcher. Nurses might opt for employment in a traditional hospital setting or somewhere else—for example, at a physician's office, a research center, or what have you. The same holds true for nurses on the night shift, though their options may be somewhat more limited than their day-shift counterparts.

 Merriam-Webster defines the word "career" as "a field for or pursuit of consecutive progressive achievement especially in public, professional, or business life" or "a profession for which one trains and which is undertaken as a permanent calling."

If your aim is to keep working nights but you want your career to advance, you can choose from several work environments, including hospitals, emergency clinics, and nursing homes (Mayo Clinic, n.d.). Specialties might include critical care nursing, emergency/trauma nursing, or neonatology nursing. Night nurses could even work in telemedicine, which involves the remote monitoring and diagnosis of patients' conditions by means of telecommunications technology. Night nurses can be involved or lead in research studies, perhaps specializing in night-time care. And of course, pursuing management positions, such as off-shift supervisor, nurse manager, department leader, or unit leader, is always an option. Table 7.1 lists a sampling of nursing employment options for night nurses.

Table 7.1: Sampling of Nursing Employment Options for Night Nurses

Role	Key Responsibility	Requirements
Evening supervisor/ house supervisor	Administrative support for clinical personnel and operations; ensure quality care	Two to three years clinical experience; one to two years' supervisory experience
Charge nurse	Support assigned unit; identify staff assignments; point person for problems and resource needs; might also have assigned patients	Usually one year clinical experience
Case manager	Coordination of patient care during transition from hospital to other facilities	One to three years clinical experience; one year case-management experience
Access coordinator	Oversee patient admissions and assignment to appropriate unit/area.	Three-plus years clinical experience
Staff nurse	Direct patient care	Depends upon specialty; most areas accept new graduates
Wellness nurse	Assist with care of elderly and supervise employees in providing care	Based on clinical experience; may be open to new nurses.
Flight nurse	Provide critical-care nursing support for patients in either air or ground transport	Three years critical-care experience
Nurse educator	Provide staff education and in-services; oversee nurses' orientation and monitor progress; support staff development	Two to three years clinical experience; knowledge of essential components of instructional development

Role	Key Responsibility	Requirements
Informatics nurse	Develop, implement, support, maintain, and evaluate electronic data and patient care documentation systems	Two years with clinical applications
Telephone support nurse	Provide patients with triage, consultation, and health care advice via phone	Three years acute-care or critical-care experience
Nurse practitioner	Provide primary care services in a clinic setting	Two years experience as NP
Faculty/ instructor	Online education for undergraduate and graduate nursing students	Five years clinical experience; one year education experience

Finding a New Job

If you're ready to find a new job, whether on day shift or night shift, we have good news for you: The U.S. Department of Labor projects much faster-than-average job growth for nurses in the immediate future. That means as employers seek to recruit and retain talented nursing staff, nurses will enjoy improved salaries, benefits, and working conditions (Isaacs, n.d.). That doesn't mean, however, that a great job will simply land at your feet. As you begin your job search, you'll want to develop a solid résumé and properly prepare for interviews.

A great place to start your job search is the ANA Nurse's Career Center (http://www.nursingworld.org/careercenter). This online resource is "designed to connect qualified nursing professionals with leading healthcare employers." As a job seeker, you can search for jobs, post a résumé, or create a search agent. Also, check out *Landing Your Perfect Nursing Job* by Lisa Mauri Thomas, published by Sigma Theta Tau International.

Developing Your Résumé

As you no doubt know, a *résumé* is simply a document used to present one's background and skills. It should contain information about the position you seek, your education, your skills, and your work experience. It should highlight contributions you've made at your various places of employment. Having a good résumé is your first step toward landing a plum new assignment. Indeed, as noted by the ANA, "It is your first chance to show yourself off to any potential employers." To develop a winning résumé, keep these points in mind (ANA, n.d.; Howell, 2009):

* **Be brief.** As noted by the ANA, "Any extra language is unnecessary and could result in a potential employer quickly losing interest." Keep the entire document under two pages—or one, if your experience is limited.
* **Be professional.** Avoid a chatty, personal tone. Also, "Don't try to be too creative with your résumé's appearance. Pink paper, cartoons, or funky fonts will get your résumé noticed—and moved to the 'do not call' pile" (Howell, 2009).
* **Don't oversell yourself.** Don't exaggerate your accomplishments; employers are sure to verify the information you give them.
* **Don't be modest.** Although you shouldn't oversell yourself, don't downplay your achievements.

* **Use "action verbs."** Highlight your achievements using action verbs, such as "develops, creates, delegates, plans, formulates, manages, serves, coordinates, directs, encourages, and collaborates" (Howell, 2009).

* **Proofread.** Check the spelling, punctuation, and grammar. Then have someone you trust do the same.

* **Highlight the skills of a night nurse.** Night staff are resourceful, often need to provide care with limited resources (compared to day shift), and are known to be good at teamwork!

Interviewing

If your résumé does its job, you'll soon find yourself landing interviews with prospective employers. Interviews, which may be conducted in person or over the phone, occur for two reasons: for the potential employer to assess whether you would be a good fit for the position and vice versa.

 If you know anyone who works for the organization where you will be interviewing, talk to that person before your interview. Try to find out what kind of personalities fit well in the job culture, whether there are any hidden expectations for employees, why employees stay with the organization, and why they leave. This will help you determine whether you will be a good fit.

Here are a few points to keep in mind to ensure your interview goes smoothly and that you put your best foot forward (Pagana, 2008):

* **Arrive early.** Drive to the location ahead of time and plan the best route. Scout out parking areas and the building entrance. On the day of the interview, allow extra time for traffic. If you find yourself running late, call your contact and notify him or

her of the situation. Try to arrive 5 to 10 minutes early so you have time to use the restroom and check your appearance.

*   **Schedule wisely.** Choose a day and time that make sense, given your work on the night shift. Don't schedule an interview for right after your shift is over or as you are waking up. You need to be clear-headed and confident!

*   **Dress appropriately.** Don't wear last night's scrubs! Be competitive in your dress and appearance. This tip is especially important for internal candidates: You want to appear as competitive for the position as external candidates.

*   **Come prepared.** Bring a folder with appropriate materials— for example, a copy of your professional license (if requested), a pad of paper or notebook and a couple of pens, and 5–10 professional-looking copies of your resume. Make sure you have reviewed the organization's website and know the organization's vision and mission. Be ready to include some facts from the website in your interview that relate to the position for which you are applying.

*   **Be positive.** Avoid making negative comments, especially about former employees, supervisors, or coworkers. Show enthusiasm.

*   **Listen.** That way, you can gather the necessary information to see if you are a good fit for the organization.

*   **Ask questions.** What skills are considered most important for success in this position? What kind of educational opportunities are offered to support career growth?

*   **Send a thank-you note.** Sending a short, handwritten note helps you stand out. Be sure to mail the note within 24 hours of the interview. Email notes are now considered appropriate, too.

If the interview is to be conducted over the phone (as is often the case in the preliminary stages of the interview process), prepare as you would for an in-person meeting. For example, you'll want to prepare a list of questions, have your resume and supporting data in front of you, and keep a pen and paper available. You may even go so far as to dress in the same clothes as you would for an in-person interview. This can help you get into "business mode" (Pagana, 2008). After the interview, you'll want to send a thank-you note, like always. Here are a few additional phone-specific tips (Pagana, 2008):

* **Control your surroundings.** Make sure there are no crying kids, barking dogs, or blaring TVs in the background.

* **Disable your phone's call-waiting option.** This prevents you from becoming distracted by incoming calls during the interview.

* **Stand up.** When you stand up, your voice sounds more confident and dynamic.

* **Smile.** Even though your interviewer won't be able to see it, he or she will be able to hear the smile in your voice. It projects a positive impression.

References

American Association of Colleges of Nursing (AACN). (2010). Your nursing career: A look at the facts. Retrieved from http://www.aacn.nche.edu/students/your-nursing-career/facts

American Nurses Association (ANA). (n.d.). Resume tips. *Nursing World.* Retrieved from http://www.nursingworld.org/careercenter/resources/ResumeTips.pdf

American Nurses Credentialing Center (ANCC). (n.d.). ANCC Certification Center. Retrieved from http://www.nursecredentialing.org/certification.aspx

Cardillo, D. (2009). Projecting your professionalism. *NSNA Imprint.* Retrieved from http://www.nsna.org/Portals/0/Skins/NSNA/pdf/Imprint_FebMar09_Feat_Cardillo.pdf

Career. (n.d.). Merriam-Webster. Retrieved from http://www.merriam-webster.com/dictionary/career

Claffey, C. (2011). How working nights can work in your favor. *American Nurse Today, 6*(11). Retrieved from http://www.americannursetoday.com/article.aspx?id=8430&fid=8364

Dracup, K. (n.d.). Master's nursing programs. *American Association of Colleges of Nursing.* Retrieved from http://www.aacn.nche.edu/education-resources/msn-article#.URbyckd2plA.aolmail

Fant, C. (n.d.). Is online nursing education right for you? *NurseTogether.* Retrieved from http://www.nursetogether.com/Education/Education-Article/itemId/1301/Is-Online-Nursing-Education-Right-for-You-.aspx

Fraser, R. (2011). *The nurse's social media advantage: How making connections and sharing ideas can enhance your nursing practice.* Indianapolis, IN: Sigma Theta Tau International.

Howell, S. (2009). Resume do's and don'ts. *Nursing, 39,* Career Directory, 20–21. Retrieved from http://journals.lww.com/nursing/fulltext/2009/01001/resume_do_s_and_don_ts.8.aspx

Isaacs, K. (n.d.). 7 best resume tips for nurses. *AllHealthcare.* Retrieved from http://allhealthcare.monster.com/careers/articles/3843-7-best-resume-tips-for-nurses?page=8

Kaiser Permanente of Colorado. (2011, June 30). SBAR technique for communication: A situational briefing model. *Institute for Healthcare Improvement.* Retrieved from www.ihi.org/knowledge/Pages/Tools/SBARTechniqueforCommunicationASituationalBriefingModel.aspx

Keefe, S. (2011). Engaging off-shift nurses. *Advance for Nurses.* Retrieved from http://nursing.advanceweb.com/Archives/Article-Archives/Engaging-Off-Shift-Nurses.aspx

Krischke, M. (2011). Exploring your nursing career options. *NurseZone.com.* Retrieved from http://www.nursezone.com/nursing-news-events/more-features/Exploring-Your-Nursing-Career-Options_38042.aspx

Kupperschmidt, B., Kientz, E., Ward, J., & Reinholz, B. (2010). A healthy work environment: It begins with you. *OJIN: The Online Journal of Issues in Nursing, 15*(1). Retrieved from http://www.nursingworld.org/MainMenuCategories/ANAMarketplace/ANAPeriodicals/OJIN/TableofContents/Vol152010/No1Jan2010/A-Healthy-Work-Environment-and-You.htm

Mayo Clinic. (n.d.). Nursing. *Mayo Clinic.* Retrieved from http://www.mayo.edu/mshs/careers/nursing

Pagana, K. (2008). *The nurse's etiquette advantage: How professional etiquette can advance your nursing career.* Indianapolis, IN: Sigma Theta Tau International.

Rothstein, M. (2012). Working as a night nurse. *Sooper Articles.* Retrieved from http://www.sooperarticles.com/health-fitness-articles/careers-articles/working-night-nurse-843625.html

Trimble, T. (n.d.). Night shift survival hints. *Emergency Nursing World.* Retrieved from http://enw.org/NightShift.htm

U.S. Department of Labor Bureau of Labor Statistics. (2012). How to become a Registered Nurse. Retrieved from http://www.bls.gov/ooh/healthcare/registered-nurses.htm#tab-4

Index

ANA Nurse's Career Center, 153
apps, for monitoring sleep, 48–49
armodafinil for alertness, 47–48
arms, exercising, 104
assessment checklist, for exercise
    level, 99
Automated Morningness-
    Eveningness Questionnaire
    (AutoMEQ), 29

B

bachelor's degrees, 144–145
balance. *See* work/life balance
bedtimes, consistency in, 30
Bennett, Michael, 8, 56, 101, 126
blood pressure, exercise and, 94
body language, 139
body mass index (BMI), calculat-
    ing, 60
Bonificio, Barbara, 105
breaks, encouraging, 121
breast cancer, 64–65
Brunt, Barbara, 42, 83, 101
BSN degrees, 144–145
Burns, Michelle J., 123

C

caffeine
    effect on sleep, 44, 46–47
    when to consume, 85
The Campaign for Nursing's
    Future website, 147
Campbell, Joseph, 133

cancer, 63–67
    exercise and, 94
cardiovascular events, 55–58
    exercise and, 93–94
career advancement
    educational opportunities,
        142–149
    job options for night-shift
        nurses, 150–152
    job searches, 152–156
    visibility at work, 134–141
Castelli, Carolyn, 124
CBT-I (cognitive behavioral
    therapy and insomnia), 46
celebrations, 118–119
Center for Nursing Renewal, 121
certification, 148–149
challenges
    comparison of shifts, 19–22
    of night shift, 8–17
change-of-shift reports, 139
Chase, Terry, 110
checklists, exercise assessment, 99
Choose My Plate paradigm, 79
circadian rhythm sleep disorders
    (CRSDs), 28
circadian rhythms
    cancer and, 64
    in sleep science, 27–29
    weight gain and, 61–62
cognitive behavioral therapy and
    insomnia (CBT-I), 46
collegiality, 118
colorectal cancer, 65–66
communication
    demonstrating skills in,
        137–141
    developing skills in, 114–115

F

family life. *See* work/life balance

fatigue
    drowsy driving, 43
    effects of, 9–12
    individual solutions, 29–34
    workplace solutions, 34–40

fertility issues, 70

financial advantages to night shift, 5

financial responsibility, 126

FitBit, 49

fitness. *See* exercise

FITT (frequency, intensity, time, and type) exercise, 98–99

Five-Factor Model for Becoming a Skilled Communicator, 114–115, 140

flexible scheduling, 116

FODMAPs, 87

food. *See also* healthful eating
    effect on sleep, 43–48
    healthy living tips, 72
    high-fiber foods, 86
    meal and snack ideas, 81
    statistics on healthful eating, 78
    weight gain and, 61–62
    what to eat, 78–80

Fraser, Robert, 140

frequency, intensity, time, and type (FITT) exercise, 98–99

G

GABA (gamma-aminobutyric acid), 45, 98

gastroesophageal reflux disease (GERD), 87

gastrointestinal problems, 63, 86–88

George, Souby, 105

GERD (gastroesophageal reflux disease), 87

glutes, exercising, 104

golfing, 97

Gonzales, Tiare Geolina, 88

grocery shopping, 80

H

Halberg, Colleen, 110

Health Insurance Portability and Accountability Act (HIPAA), 141

health issues
    cancer, 63–67
    cardiovascular events, 55–58
    challenges of night shift, 12–13, 54–55
    diabetes, 58–60
    gastrointestinal problems, 86–88
    obesity, 60–63
    reproductive issues, 70
    stress, 67–69
    tips for healthy living, 70–73

healthful eating. *See also* food
    meal and snack ideas, 81
    statistics, 78
    what to eat, 78–80
    workplace tips, 82–86

X–Y–Z